Direct-to-Consumer Testing: The Role of Laboratory Medicine

Editors

NICOLE V. TOLAN
ROBERT D. NERENZ

CLINICS IN LABORATORY MEDICINE

www.labmed.theclinics.com

Editor-in-Chief

MILENKO JOVAN TANASIJEVIC

March 2020 • Volume 40 • Number 1

ELSEVIER

1600 John F. Kennedy Boulevard • Suite 1800 • Philadelphia, Pennsylvania, 19103-2899

http://www.theclinics.com

CLINICS IN LABORATORY MEDICINE Volume 40, Number 1
March 2020 ISSN 0272-2712, ISBN-13: 978-0-323-75444-6

Editor: Katerina Heidhausen
Developmental Editor: Laura Fisher

Reprints. For copies of 100 or more, of articles in this publication, please contact the Commercial Reprints Department, Elsevier Inc., 360 Park Avenue South, New York, New York 10010-1710. Tel. 212-633-3874, Fax: 212-633-3820, E-mail: reprints@elsevier.com.

Clinics in Laboratory Medicine (ISSN 0272-2712) is published quarterly by Elsevier Inc., 360 Park Avenue South, New York, NY 10010-1710. Months of issue are March, June, September, and December. Business and Editorial offices: 1600 John F. Kennedy Blvd., Suite 1800, Philadelphia, PA 19103-2899. Periodicals postage paid at NewYork, NY and additional mailing offices. Subscription prices are $277.00 per year (US individuals), $571.00 per year (US institutions), $100.00 per year (US students), $349.00 per year (Canadian individuals), $693.00 per year (Canadian institutions), $100.00 per year (Canadian students), $404.00 per year (international individuals), $693.00 per year (international institutions), $185.00 (international students). Foreign air speed delivery is included in all Clinics subscription prices. All prices are subject to change without notice. POSTMASTER: Send address changes to *Clinics in Laboratory Medicine,* Elsevier Health Sciences Division, Subscription Customer Service, 3251 Riverport Lane, Maryland Heights, MO 63043. **Customer Service: 1-800-654-2452 (US). From outside of the US and Canada, call 1-314-447-8871. Fax: 1-314-447-8029. E-mail: journalscustomerservice-usa@elsevier.com (for print support) or journalsonlinesupport-usa@elsevier.com (for online support).**

Clinics in Laboratory Medicine is covered in *EMBASE/Exerpta Medica, MEDLINE/PubMed (Index Medicus),* Cinahl, *Current Contents/Clinical Medicine, BIOSIS* and *ISI/BIOMED.*

Contributors

EDITOR-IN-CHIEF

MILENKO JOVAN TANASIJEVIC, MD, MBA
Vice Chair for Clinical Pathology and Quality, Department of Pathology, Director of Clinical Laboratories, Brigham and Women's Hospital, Dana-Farber Cancer Institute, Associate Professor of Pathology, Harvard Medical School, Boston, Massachusetts, USA

EDITORS

NICOLE V. TOLAN, PhD, DABCC
Assistant Professor of Pathology, Harvard Medical School, Medical Director, POCT and Associate Medical Director, Clinical Chemistry, Brigham and Women's Hospital, Boston, Massachusetts, USA

ROBERT D. NERENZ, PhD, DABCC
Assistant Professor of Pathology and Laboratory Medicine, Geisel School of Medicine at Dartmouth, Assistant Director of Clinical Chemistry, Dartmouth-Hitchcock Medical Center, Lebanon, New Hampshire, USA

AUTHORS

NIKOLA A. BAUMANN, PhD, DABCC
Co-Director of the Central Clinical Lab and Central Processing, Assistant Professor, Department of Laboratory Medicine and Pathology, Mayo Clinic, Rochester, Minnesota, USA

MELISSA M. BUDELIER, PhD
Fellow, Department of Pathology and Immunology, Washington University School of Medicine, St Louis, Missouri, USA

CHRISTIAN DAMEFF, MD
Departments of Emergency Medicine, Biomedical Informatics, Computer Science and Engineering, University of California, San Diego, La Jolla, California, USA

MARY BETH PALKO DINULOS, MD
Associate Professor of Pediatrics and Pathology, The Geisel School of Medicine at Dartmouth, Section Chief, Genetics and Child Development, Dartmouth-Hitchcock Medical Center, Lebanon, New Hampshire, USA

KORNELIA D. GALIOR, PhD, DABCC
Associate Director of Clinical Chemistry, Assistant Professor, Department of Pathology and Laboratory Medicine, University of Wisconsin School of Medicine and Public Health, Madison, Wisconsin, USA

EMILY L. GILL, PhD
Department of Pathology and Laboratory Medicine, Children's Hospital of Philadelphia, Philadelphia, Pennsylvania, USA

ANN M. GRONOWSKI, PhD
Professor, Department of Pathology and Immunology, Washington University School of Medicine, St Louis, Missouri, USA

DANIEL T. HOLMES, MD, FCRCP
Professor, Department of Pathology and Laboratory Medicine, St. Paul's Hospital, Department of Pathology and Laboratory Medicine, University of British Columbia, Vancouver, British Columbia, Canada

TIMOTHY SCOTT ISBELL, PhD, DABCC, FAACC
Department of Pathology, Division of Clinical Pathology, Saint Louis University School of Medicine, St Louis, Missouri, USA

JOEL A. LEFFERTS, PhD
Assistant Director and Assistant Professor, Clinical Genomics and Advanced Technology Laboratory, Department of Pathology and Laboratory Medicine, Dartmouth-Hitchcock Medical Center, Geisel School of Medicine at Dartmouth, Lebanon, New Hampshire, USA

CHRISTOPHER A. LONGHURST, MD
Departments of Medicine and Pediatrics, University of California, San Diego, La Jolla, California, USA

STEPHEN R. MASTER, MD, PhD
Chief, Division of Laboratory Medicine, Director, Michael Palmieri Laboratory for Metabolic and Advanced Diagnostics, Children's Hospital of Philadelphia, Associate Professor of Pathology and Laboratory Medicine, Perelman School of Medicine, University of Pennsylvania, Philadelphia, Pennsylvania, USA

LAUREN M. PETERSEN, PhD
Molecular Diagnostics Fellow (Clinical Genomics and Advanced Technology Laboratory), Department of Pathology and Laboratory Medicine, Dartmouth-Hitchcock Medical Center, Lebanon, New Hampshire, USA

NICOLE V. TOLAN, PhD, DABCC
Assistant Professor of Pathology, Harvard Medical School, Medical Director, POCT and Associate Medical Director, Clinical Chemistry, Brigham and Women's Hospital, Boston, Massachusetts, USA

JEFFREY TULLY, MD
Department of Anesthesiology and Pain Medicine, UC Davis Medical Center, Sacramento, California, USA

STEPHANIE E. VALLEE, MS
Section of Genetics and Child Development, Department of Pediatrics, Dartmouth-Hitchcock Medical Center, Lebanon, New Hampshire, USA

Contents

With the ever-increasing market share of direct-to-consumer (DTC) testing, projected to surpass $350 million this year, health care professionals must address the health literacy gap that exists between what the clinician knows and what the general public understands about clinical laboratory testing. Health literacy is lowest among people with lower socioeconomic status and results in poorer outcomes. However, these individuals represent those that would benefit most from valuable DTC testing. There is a need for unbiased and universally accessible tools to help improve consumers' understanding of test utility, limitations to the accuracy of results, and result interpretation.

Debate exists between the consumer and the health care provider when it comes to the value of direct-to-consumer (DTC) testing. At the heart of the issue is the observation that consumers are identifying value in DTC testing as evidenced by an expanding market, and health care providers are skeptical of their value from an analytical and clinical utility perspective. The aim of this article is to briefly review the subject of DTC testing with a specific focus on value from the perspective of the consumer and the health care provider.

Companies that offer direct-to-consumer (DTC) testing on specimens such as saliva, blood, or urine, allow consumers to order laboratory tests without the involvement of a health care provider. This approach allows individuals to have direct access to their own laboratory results, interpret them, and make decisions regarding their health care. However, as with conventional clinical laboratory testing, there are factors that will impact the accuracy of DTC test results and limitations that consumers need to be aware of. This article focuses on challenges with DTC testing specifically related to preanalytical errors, result reporting, and result interpretation.

quality, and increase clinician efficiency. Wearables have significant potential to achieve these goals but are currently limited by lack of widespread integrations into electronic health records, biosensor data collection types, and a lack of scientifically rigorous literature showing benefit.

The number of companies offering direct-to-consumer (DTC) genetic tests is increasing. There is growing concern over whether DTC genetic companies should be allowed to offer clinically relevant testing that has only been possible under medical care. DTC genetic testing can be incomplete, inaccurate, and inappropriate. The usefulness of such testing is extremely limited and it is unclear how well customers understand reported results. Research on the long-term impact of DTC genetic testing is necessary to determine if stricter regulations regarding the performance of DTC genetic testing are necessary.

Direct-to-consumer (DTC) laboratory testing is a rapidly growing industry. However, the idea of consumers ordering their own laboratory tests has raised ethical concerns. Respect for autonomy, beneficence, nonmaleficence, and justice are core principles of biomedical ethics. Although DTC testing would seem to offer autonomy to consumers, autonomy is only maintained if certain criteria are met, including intentionality, understanding, and noncontrol. There is little published evidence to support either beneficence or maleficence of DTC testing. Finally, there are conflicting opinions about the justice of DTC testing and whether it increases or decreases health disparities.

This article provides a brief introduction to some of the challenges associated with DTC testing, including: the concerns for overall limited healthcare value and unsubstantiated excessive monitoring of health and wellness markers, risks for reduced test quality from DTC testing companies claiming regulatory exemption, the impact of communication breakdown with a qualified healthcare professional leading to unnecessary worry and inappropriate self-management, and the downstream effects DTC testing has placed on our already overburdened healthcare system.

CLINICS IN LABORATORY MEDICINE

SERIES OF RELATED INTEREST

Surgical Pathology Clinics
Available at: https://www.surgpath.theclinics.com/

THE CLINICS ARE NOW AVAILABLE ONLINE!
Access your subscription at:
www.theclinics.com

Preface

Direct–to-Consumer Testing: The Role of Laboratory Medicine Physicians and Scientists

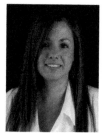 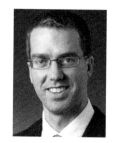

Nicole V. Tolan, PhD, DABCC   Robert D. Nerenz, PhD, DABCC
Editors

We've seen the consumer-driven laboratory testing market grow at an exponential rate as companies offer an increasing number and variety of recreational genetic testing, oncogene panels, mail-in laboratory testing, at-home point-of-care tests, and wearable devices. Direct-to-consumer (DTC) testing is marketed to consumers with very different motivations ranging from simple entertainment to the early identification or monitoring of disease. As individuals become increasingly engaged in their own health care, DTC testing represents an extension of our current system with the potential for many benefits, especially for those without access to traditional medical care or healthcare coverage.

However, while most consumers want to take control of their own health, most do not have sufficient health literacy to understand the implications of testing or to interpret their results. Can nonmedically trained consumers be expected to understand the performance characteristics of DTC tests, particularly those intended to determine an individual's susceptibility to hereditary cancers or other inherited conditions? Should consent be required from family members who may be affected by a relative's genetic DTC test results?

While there is substantial public support for "on-demand" clinical laboratory testing and increased ownership of an individual's test results, many are concerned about the potential to cause harm. Are DTC testing companies providing analytically valid results with sufficient interpretation and medical guidance? Will the results be followed up appropriately by consumers? Is it even ethical to allow access to any test at any time, regardless of medical necessity?

Many challenges exist from the perspective of clinical providers, namely, laboratory physicians and scientists. What is the role of the clinical laboratorian in this rapidly

Clin Lab Med 40 (2020) ix–x
https://doi.org/10.1016/j.cll.2019.12.002
0272-2712/20/© 2019 Published by Elsevier Inc.

evolving field and how can we integrate ourselves into the process to maximize benefit and minimize harm? Will care providers become inundated with requests to review DTC results that may indicate risk for disease but are not clinically confirmed or significant? Furthermore, without clear communication of results, it may be more challenging for physicians to manage their patients, report communicable diseases, and follow up with critical results.

As DTC testing is still in its infancy, many of these questions have yet to be definitively answered. This collection of articles by prominent clinical professionals addresses core concepts of DTC testing from the clinical perspective, with a detailed discussion of potential benefits, limitations, and challenges.

Nicole V. Tolan, PhD, DABCC
Department of Pathology
Harvard Medical School
Brigham and Women's Hospital
75 Francis Street, Cotran 2
Boston, MA 02115, USA

Robert D. Nerenz, PhD, DABCC
Geisel School of Medicine at Dartmouth
Dartmouth-Hitchcock Medical Center
Department of Pathology and
Laboratory Medicine
1 Medical Center Drive
Lebanon, NH 03756, USA

E-mail addresses:
ntolan@bwh.harvard.edu (N.V. Tolan)
robert.d.nerenz@hitchcock.org (R.D. Nerenz)

Health Literacy and the Desire to Manage One's Own Health

Nicole V. Tolan, PhD, DABCC

KEYWORDS

- Direct-to-consumer testing • Health literacy • Health information • Health disparities
- Laboratory medicine • Clinical laboratorians

KEY POINTS

- Consumers are turning to direct-to-consumer (DTC) testing because it is easily accessible, affordable, and they are dissatisfied with long waits, short appointments, and inadequate control of their health care management in the current health care system.
- Those who may benefit the most from inexpensive, on-demand, and clinically actionable DTC testing are the least likely to have sufficient health literacy to be able to use and interpret these tests correctly.
- Laboratory professionals play a critical role in providing education to consumers and health care providers while also doing their part to ensure that DTC testing is ethical, easily understood by consumers, accurate, and of high quality.

INTRODUCTION

With health care spending at an all-time high, attention has focused on reducing the total cost by eliminating unnecessary laboratory testing and low-value screening. However, despite these efforts, some clinicians have proposed a perhaps perplexing solution: direct-to-consumer (DTC) testing. DTC testing does not require a physician's order, or the cost of seeing a provider, and offers substantially decreased costs to patients with high-deductible insurance plans or the 27.5 million people in the United States who were without coverage in 2018.[1] DTC testing offers the potential of providing an increased health economic value through improved outcomes by identifying disease earlier or more routinely monitoring chronic conditions.

DTC testing could represent a component of the patient-centered health care model, which we know results in better outcomes, increased patient satisfaction, and therapy compliance. Further, as health care providers and policy makers incentivize preventive health care and move away from the focus of disease management,

Department of Pathology, Harvard Medical School, Brigham and Women's Hospital, 75 Francis Street, Cotran 2, Boston, MA 02115, USA
E-mail address: ntolan@bwh.harvard.edu

Clin Lab Med 40 (2020) 1–12
https://doi.org/10.1016/j.cll.2019.11.007
0272-2712/20/© 2019 Elsevier Inc. All rights reserved.

DTC testing offers an enticing approach to more frequent monitoring of overall health and wellness. In this regard, DTC testing supports patients who seek medical treatment sooner, potentially avoiding complications associated with the progression of disease. DTC testing disrupts the traditional models of health care and empowers consumers to take charge of their own health.

Thus, in theory, DTC testing could lead to an ultimate reduction in overall health care costs.

However, there is a need for unbiased and universally accessible tools to help improve consumers' understanding of test utility, limitations to the accuracy of results, and result interpretation.

DESIRE TO MANAGE OWN HEALTH

Patients believe health and wellness monitoring is beneficial and they are willing to pay out of pocket for it. Despite the low or lacking value of many DTC tests[2] and concerns for inaccuracy of results,[3–5] consumers desire the ability to order their own tests to monitor their wellness and to detect disease sooner. Although there is great debate on the benefit and potential consequences of wellness testing, because overtesting can also lead to false results and unnecessary follow-up testing and medical care,[4] consumers find great value in the perceived ability to manage their health through DTC testing.

Further, DTC testing has been positioned as a key element in increasing the general populations' engagement with managing their own health care.[6] According to the 2015 *Self-Care in Today's Changing Healthcare Environment* survey conducted by Ipsos in collaboration with the National Council on Patient Information Education (NCPIE) and Pfizer,[7] consumers are taking a more active role in their health management. Most respondents believe they are capable of taking control of their own health and they know where to find answers to their health questions.

The two core principles outlined by the US Department of Health and Human Services, Office of Disease Prevention and Health Promotion pertaining to the communication of health information to the general public are (1) all people have the right to health information that helps them make informed health decisions; and (2) health services should be delivered in ways that are easy to understand and that improve health, longevity, and quality of life.[8]

However, most Americans are unable to comprehend much of the health information presented in health care facilities, retail outlets, in general media, and throughout their communities. It was estimated that nearly 90% of Americans had challenges using health information that was generally available[9–11] more than a decade ago; this percentage is likely even higher now considering the increased complexity of current health information.

HEALTH LITERACY AND DIRECT-TO-CONSUMER TESTING

Although most participants in the Ipsos survey[7] were confident in their abilities to manage their health, opponents to DTC testing are concerned that most consumers are unaware of the limitations of laboratory testing, in general, and neither have sufficient knowledge to interpret test results nor can they make informed decisions about their health with this information.[12–14] Studies of health care portals indicate that laboratory reports are one of the top three sections in the electronic medical record that are least understood and result in patients seeking additional information on the Internet to better understand their results.[15] Laboratory testing results place a high reading and numeracy burden on consumers, and nearly 50% are unable even to determine whether results are normal or abnormal.[16] Even with a clinical health care provider as part of the laboratory testing process, approximately 34% of patients have unanswered questions about their laboratory tests.[17]

As shown in **Fig. 1**, there are several advantages and disadvantages across the continuum of the various models of clinical testing. Although clinical laboratory testing offers the highest-quality, evidence-based diagnostic testing, it also requires time to transport, receive, and process samples. Point-of-care and near-patient testing offer the advantages of more rapid turnaround time and supporting patient-physician interaction alongside testing, but most individuals performing the test are not scientifically trained and their main focus is on patient care. DTC testing offers increased access to testing at low out-of-pocket costs, without health insurance coverage. However, concerns remain on the impact of limited consumer health literacy and the inability to recognize and prevent confounders to test accuracy. Proponents believe the DTC testing model will benefit from increased consumer involvement in their health care management, whereas concerns remain on the impact of limited consumer health literacy, and the inability to recognize and prevent confounders to test accuracy. Although DTC testing offers the privacy consumers desire, this can also lead to gaps in communication. These limitations can be overcome with the involvement of a health care professional through telemedicine and medical consultation, but requires redefining the DTC testing model.

Despite the average reading level of the US population at the eighth to ninth grade and that 20% of the population reads at the fifth grade level, most medical material and reports are written at or above the 10th grade level[18] because they have historically been intended for interpretation by medical professionals. According to the US

Models of Clinical Testing

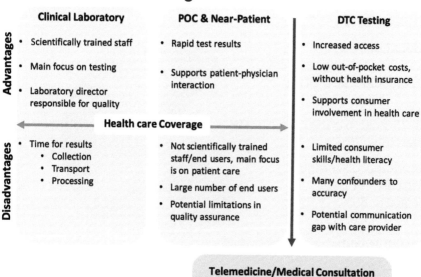

Fig. 1. The advantages and disadvantages across the continuum of various models of clinical testing. ED, emergency department. UC, urgent care.

Department of Health and Human Series (HHS) Office of Disease Prevention and Health Promotion, based on the National Assessment of Adult Literacy (NAAL) survey, only 12% of US adults have proficient health literacy, defined as "the ability to obtain, process, and understand basic health information and services to make appropriate health decisions."[10,12] With 35% of the US population (77 million adults in 2003) having basic or below-basic health literacy, these individuals currently have limitations in understanding and following medical information intended for the general public and prescription instructions.

However, overall health literacy is lower in individuals with a myriad of complex, interdependent factors contributing to their lower socioeconomic status:[10] race, education, age, insurance coverage, self-assessment of overall health, occupation, and income (**Fig. 2**). Consequently, those who may benefit the most from inexpensive, on-demand, and clinically actionable DTC testing are the least likely to have sufficient health literacy to be able to use and interpret these tests correctly. Lower health literacy disproportionately affects those of lower socioeconomic status and minority groups, predisposing them to an increased likelihood of missing necessary medical tests, higher rates of emergency department visits, and poor overall management of chronic diseases such as diabetes and high blood pressure.[9,19]

Are consumers knowledgeable enough to order the right test, understand and follow the test instructions correctly, interpret their results, and know when additional follow-up is necessary?

Basic/Below Basic Health Literacy in United States: 35%

Race
Black: 57%
Hispanic: 65%

Education
Less than HS degree: 76%
HS graduate/GED: 44%

Age
65–75 y old: 51%
Over 75 y: 70%

Insurance Coverage
Medicare: 57%
Medicaid: 60%
No insurance: 53%

Overall Health
Poor: 69%
Fair: 63%

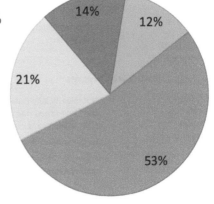

■ Proficient ■ Intermediate ■ Basic ■ Below Basic

Fig. 2. Socioeconomic variables and corresponding health literacy. The 2003 National Assessment of Adult Literacy was administered to approximately 19,000 adults, of whom 35% were determined to have basic or below-basic health literacy. The percentages of survey respondents with basic or below-basic literacy are shown for each variable associated with lower socioeconomic status: race, education, age, insurance coverage, and self-assessment of overall health. HS, high school; GED, general education diploma.

Several examples exist in the history of DTC testing and demonstrate that consumers are generally unaware of:

1. **Test utility and indications for use:** several DTC tests currently on the market are of limited utility,[2] and although the Federal Trade Commission (FTC) is charged with ensuring against (overtly) false claims and deceptive marketing practices, the resources to police the vast DTC testing market would have to be substantial to ensure compliance. Further, it is increasingly difficult to differentiate between DTC and direct-access testing (DAT), adding to the complexity of managing this space. This testing is commonly performed using in vitro diagnostic assays in the same hospital and commercial laboratories as medical testing that is ordered by a physician, but is ordered directly by patients without consultation.[20,21] In reality, there are only a limited number of tests that are indicated for generalized screening (eg, lipid profile) and consumers may not be aware of the pretest probability necessary for accurate and actionable results of those developed to predict disease.

2. **Limitations of the test:** at-home pregnancy tests offer a prime example, in that many consumers are not aware that various factors should be considered to ensure the optimal performance of the test:
   - Storage requirements of the test device
   - The effect of analytical time on results, reading the test too early/late
   - Limit of detection and effect of urine concentration
   - Various forms of human chorionic gonadotropin detected/not detected
   - The requirement for quality control acceptability for test validity

3. **How to interpret results:** both genetic and nongenetic DTC tests have been shown to have ineffective result reporting for the general public. For genetic testing in particular, the limitations of the algorithms used to calculate lifetime genetic risk were not well understood or apparent to consumers, leading to poor consumer recognition of the predictive limitations of these tests.[22]

4. **When follow-up testing is required:** patients often struggle to differentiate a normal from nonnormal result,[16] but, even more sophisticated, when follow-up testing may (or may not) be required for results outside the reference interval.[14] In an attempt to overcome this limitation, an increasing number of DTC testing companies are providing results in personalized reports or with board-certified physicians or nurses to aid consumers in their result interpretation.

Inability of the general public to order tests correctly and understand their limitations is a major factor challenging medical professionals in supporting the model of DTC testing. Highly trained health care professionals are capable of interpreting laboratory testing results; perhaps they are even aware of the limitations of the assay and its performance. They consider the results in the context of the patient's medical history and symptoms; all these considerations were likely made even before ordering the test. However, given the limited basic medical knowledge and health literacy of the general public, these considerations are likely absent, with downstream sequelae that can have serious ramifications for these consumers and the already overtaxed health care system with increasing unnecessary follow-up.[23,24]

Although DTC testing offers the privacy consumers desire, this can also lead to gaps in communication. However many individuals are taking their DTC testing results to their physicians, there are a multitude of others who are not and may not be getting the medical attention/treatment they need based on their results.[25,26] These limitations can be overcome with the involvement of a health care professional through telemedicine and medical consultation, but this would require redefining the current DTC testing model.

"Genetic data are the most personal of data" and represent a unique identifier to individuals and their biological relatives that is inherently identifiable.[27] However, 80% of consumers who order genetics testing participate in genetic research, allowing these data to feed therapeutics development. From 2008 to 2013, 23andMe mapped the genome of nearly 500,000 people. Roughly 26 million people have performed DTC genetic ancestry testing, which is expected to grow to more than 100 million in the next few years.[28] Variations in the privacy procedures and policies of DTC testing companies make it challenging for consumers to fully comprehend how their data can be used, and even sold to third parties. In the present era of immediate digital consent, many consumers are simply agreeing to these policies in order to perform DTC testing without reading the fine print, similar to the operating system upgrade agreements periodically pushed to mobile devices.

In addition, a growing number of consumers are choosing to voluntarily share their results with companies that offer interpretative services, from raw genetic data or results from continuous health monitors, without fully understanding the potential consequences for themselves and their biological relatives, now or in the future.[29] Concerns for data security are ever increasing, especially considering that even protected health information is inadvertently shared,[30] which extends to the genetic testing of minors; many, but not all, states restrict surreptitious testing in an effort to protect the rights of youth.

Akin to DTC pharmaceutical drug marketing in the United States, many think DTC testing companies are appealing to the fears of underlying conditions/diseases, which is only possible because of the limited health literacy of most Americans.[31] Many policy makers and health care professionals have advocated for increased consumer education pertaining to the potential risks of DTC testing, including the risk of falling prey to fraudulent claims and deceptive marketing as well as ordering tests that offer little to no value in medical outcomes or overall health.[2,6,32,33]

Fraud charges were recently issued against several companies targeting individuals 65 years of age and older, offering, at no cost to them, genetic testing to estimate cancer risk or as part of a pharmacogenetic assessment.[34] In what has been one of the largest health care fraud schemes, laboratories were paying illegal kickbacks and bribes to medical professionals who were working with fraudulent telemarketers in exchange for the referral of Medicare beneficiaries. These seniors were subjected to aggressive scare tactics, such as telling patients that if they did not have the testing performed, they could have a variety of fatal conditions. Often the laboratory tests were ordered by one of the company physicians "And these doctors, in many cases, have zero contact with the patient and no knowledge of their health care situation or needs," said Joe Beemsterboer, Senior Deputy Chief of the fraud section in the Criminal Division of the Department of Justice. Even worse, the laboratory was not always reporting the results, and when it did, it did not include any medical consultation to interpret the results, providing no meaningful information. This fraudulent activity was detected through traceable, illegal Medicare billing practices and perhaps represents only a small fraction of similar practices that are undetected because of the nature of DTC testing charging individual consumers directly.

BRIDGING THE GAP: HEALTH INFORMATION AND HEALTH LITERACY

Basic health literacy is fundamental to helping people follow medical recommendations. The previous Assistant Secretary for Health, Dr Howard K. Koh, highlights that health literacy needs to be made a public health priority, as an essential component of the success for the national health agenda, stating, "The responsibility is ours as health professions to communicate in plain language."[8] Doing this requires filling the gap between what health care professionals know and what the general public understands, starting first with the youngest generations.

As the most fundamental of examples, whole-blood glucose consumer testing in the diabetic population has been shown to successfully improve outcomes by allowing consumers to titrate insulin dosing more stringently. However, this easily understood condition, and straightforward monitoring, also took time and education of the general public on the part of health care professionals.[35]

The HHS Office of Disease Prevention and Health Promotion has outlined 7 goals to improve health literacy:

1. Develop and disseminate health and safety information that is accurate, accessible, and actionable
2. Promote changes in the health care system that improve health information, communication, informed decision making, and access to health services
3. Incorporate accurate, standards-based, and developmentally appropriate health and science information and curricula in childcare and education through the university level
4. Support and expand local efforts to provide adult education, English language instruction, and culturally and linguistically appropriate health information services in the community
5. Build partnerships, develop guidance, and change policies
6. Increase basic research and the development, implementation, and evaluation of practices and interventions to improve health literacy
7. Increase the dissemination and use of evidence-based health literacy practices and interventions

The 2004 Institute of Medicine report outlines the framework for improving health literacy[9] by improving background medical knowledge, general health language, and communication skills. However, these strategies are limited in how to specifically address the general public's health literacy pertaining to clinical testing information, an area that has been shown to pose serious challenges for general health consumers but is a fundamental component of overall health care management.

What are some of the essential components to increasing health literacy, specifically for the specialty of clinical testing?

Based on the strategies outlined by HHS in response to the NAAL survey[12] and clinical laboratory experts,[36] there are 5 key areas to close the gap between the health information currently available and the health literacy of the general public.

Identify Key Stakeholders

Starting by advocating for federal programs to increase health literacy with those in particular positions of influence (governmental policy makers and lobbyists, health care administrators and providers, educators and students) is essential to establish health literacy standards. Addressing this as a disparities initiative with full governmental backing and focus on health inequities in the general population would allow further buy-in and engagement of relevant parties.

In addition, setting national standards on health education for primary through university core education, starting with the youngest generations, will build a general population capable of navigating this new health care paradigm. By also including training for health care providers to better communicate complex health information, consumers and providers will communicate more effectively.

Standardization of Consumer-Facing Medical and Laboratory Information

Aside from oversight by the FTC in the United States, ensuring against faulty or misleading claims, there is little oversight or standardization in how DTC materials and tests reports provide medical information. Further, because 88% of survey respondents have less than proficient health literacy,[12] reports need to be designed accordingly.

With a systems approach, laboratory testing information and informational health resources intended for the general public can be designed to be universally accessible, cultural and linguistic considerations can be made, and guidelines can be developed. Much like the universal access requirements for buildings and telecommunications, clinical laboratory information pertaining to DTC testing must be expected to meet specific requirements, with these requirements tied to public and private funding. It is essential that laboratory professionals lead this effort because the most common use of health record portals is to review laboratory testing data, which shows the focus on clinical laboratory data in consumer health management.

As a larger initiative to improve health literacy, public insurers alongside clinical laboratorians could develop exemplary health information materials. Although not specifically directed at DTC testing, this work would benefit Medicare and Medicaid beneficiaries in understanding their health, but would also provide models for DTC testing companies to meet the guidelines for laboratory information access and design mentioned earlier.

The first step is to agree that guidelines are necessary; the second is to define what constitutes accessible health information and make it widely known.

Provide Accessible, High-Quality Information

The standard design for clinical laboratory health information intended for the general public must reduce overall health literacy demands and meet consumer expectations. Information must be in appropriate language and sophistication for consumers but also for health care providers as a guide for advising their patients who are performing DTC testing. This requirement means that DTC testing companies must disclose sufficient information about their products and services and provide clear, developmentally appropriate:

- Evidence-based explanation of test indications for use (screening, diagnosis, prognosis, disease monitoring), including the population to be tested
- Benefits and limitations of testing, considering the pretest probability for optimal test performance
- Instructions for performing the test, including preanalytical considerations from pretest preparation (eg, fasting) to test and sample handling requirements
- Information on what method is used for testing and its performance characteristics (akin to reporting requirements for tumor marker monitoring)
- Clear and understandable test results, including the description of normal reference intervals and the significance of results
- Sufficient interpretative information, based on unbiased evidence, to aid in health care management decisions, as well as reputable resources for additional information

- Information about any follow-up testing that may be required and prominent instructions to contact a qualified health care provider with any questions or concerns

Clinical laboratory physicians and scientists are the only medical professionals trained in the technical and clinical aspects of laboratory testing and are uniquely positioned to help provide thorough and evidence-based information pertaining to DTC testing. In this, a classification strategy assessing the value of DTC tests should be made available to the general public, outlining what test could improve health and which provide no valuable health information. Critical assessment of DTC tests available on the market is needed in an accessible format.[2] As pertains to wellness monitoring, additional studies are required and should be performed by these experts to determine the reasonable intervals for repeat testing, based on outcomes and overall improvements in morbidity and mortality.

Routes to Informational Resources

It is essential that health care providers distribute understandable materials about DTC testing to consumers because this is one of the most important sources of health information for all health literacy levels.[12] Physicians play a key role in disseminating reliable information and ensuring that it is accessible to all of their patients.

However, reaching those with health disparities, particularly those without health insurance, means that multiple sources for information must be provided. Serious consideration for the general media to increase health literacy, and for providing health information to the public, must be made. The NAAL[12] survey indicated that adults at the below-basic health literacy level were the least likely to use any written material to obtain information on health topics, and general media may be the best route to reach this health literacy group.

Maintaining the Involvement of Appropriate Clinical Health Care Professionals

Including a trained health care professional in the process of DTC testing is essential to the success of the system, enabling improved outcomes and reducing total health care costs. Genetic counselors play an important role in helping consumers understand their genetic testing results. Their education, training, and patient consultation cannot simply be replaced by automated interpretative services online. The same is true for primary care providers and laboratory medicine consultants. The need to connect consumers with appropriate health care professionals to aid in test interpretation and health care decisions should be a major priority.

Increased engagement with the public to share clinical and laboratory knowledge, increase recognition of the expertise of clinical laboratorians, and to learn more about the public's expectation of DTC testing is necessary to drive culture change and improve overall health literacy.

Many DTC testing companies are using medical doctors to place orders and answer questions (who may also be holding the laboratory's Clinical Laboratory Improvement Amendments [CLIA] certificate), but many have limited clinical laboratory specialty and technical knowledge. This gap points to the need for laboratory medicine professionals to assist with the selection of the most appropriate tests, clarifying results, and detailing additional testing that may be required.

SUMMARY

Consumers are turning to DTC testing because it is easily accessible, affordable, and they are dissatisfied with long waits, short appointments, and inadequate control of their health care management in the current health care system. Patients are increasingly moving toward health care models that prioritize health and wellness in the hopes of preventing disease and optimizing health. Given the unhindered growth of DTC testing, laboratory professionals play a critical role in providing education to consumers and health care providers while also doing their part to ensure that DTC testing is ethical, easily understood by consumers, accurate, and of high quality.

Well-performing tests with good analytical and diagnostic performance for which the preanalytical limitations can be overcome or can be collected at regulated phlebotomy sites, that are performed in CLIA-certified laboratories, have the potential to prove their benefit and overcome several limitations to the traditional health care system. The ability to monitor chronic diseases and appropriately screen for disease or infection, more frequently, faster, more conveniently, and at a reduced cost/charge to the patients, offers a beneficial dynamic to the larger health care delivery model. However, DTC companies should be mandated to perform to the same quality standards as traditional clinical laboratories and bear the burden of proof for the diagnostics information their testing claims to provide.

Health literacy is lowest among people with lower socioeconomic status and this results in poorer outcomes. However, these individuals stand to receive the most benefit from clinically valuable DTC testing. Because trained health care providers do not necessarily assist in the interpretation of DTC testing results, these companies must provide developmentally appropriate reports, comprehensible by their targeted consumers. In order for DTC testing to be advantageous, the general public must also be able to adequately understand the clinical utility of testing and be able to interpret the meaning of their results.

A multidisciplinary approach to addressing health literacy disparities, specifically as they pertain to clinical laboratory health information, is essential to supporting the public's use of DTC testing as a safe and effective contribution to modern health care. Otherwise, DTC testing will continue to enable unnecessary testing that increases health care spending with unnecessary follow-up and burdens the already strained health care system.

DISCLOSURE

The author has nothing to disclose.

REFERENCES

1. Berchick ER, Barnett JC, Upton RD. Current population reports, health insurance coverage in the United States: 2018. US Census Bureau, Department of Commerce; 2019. p. 60–267. Available at. https://www.census.gov/library/publications/2019/demo/p60-267.html. Accessed November 16, 2019.
2. Lovett KM, Mackey TK, Liang BA. Evaluating the evidence: direct-to-consumer screening tests advertised online. J Med Screen 2012;19:141–53.
3. Kaufman DJ, Bollinger JM, Dvoskin RL, et al. Risky business: risk perception and the use of medical services among customers of DTC personal genetic testing. J Genet Couns 2012;21:413–22.
4. Ioannidis JPA. Stealth research and theranos: reflections and update 1 year later. JAMA 2016;316:389–90.
5. Riley J, Stoll K. Blurred lines: comparing direct-to-consumer and clinical testing. Washington, DC: Clinical Laboratory News, American Association of Clinical Chemistry; 2019. Available at: https://www.aacc.org/publications/cln/articles/2019/julyaug/blurred-lines. Accessed August 1, 2019.

6. American Association for Clinical Chemistry. Position statement: direct-to-consumer laboratory testing. 2015. Available at: https://www.aacc.org/-/media/Files/Health-and-Science-Policy/Position-Statements/DirecttoConsumerLaboratoryTesting.pdf?la=en&hash=18864E273BDECF27DFE2F3305E21422AD1BB8A22.   Accessed August 1, 2019.

7. Ipsos, National Council on Patient Information and Education and Pfizer. Self-Care in Today's Changing Healthcare Environment. 2014. Available at: http://www.bemedwise.org/docs/resources/ohs_sc_survey_infographic.pdf. Accessed August 1, 2019.

8. U.S. Department of Health and Human Services, Office of Disease Prevention and Health Promotion. National action plan to improve health literacy. 2010. Available at: https://health.gov/communication/initiatives/health-literacy-action-plan.asp. Accessed August 1, 2019.

9. Nielsen-Bohlman L, Panzer AM, Kindig DA. Institute of Medicine Committee on Health. Health Literacy: A Prescription to End Confusion. Washington, DC: National Academies Press; 2004.

10. Kutner M, Greenberg E, Jin Y, et al. The health literacy of America's adults: results from the 2003 National Assessment of Adult Literacy (NCES 2006-483). Washington, DC: U.S. Department of Education, National Center for Education Statistics; 2006.

11. Rudd R, Anderson J, Oppenheimer S, et al. Health literacy: an update of public health and medical literature. Review of adult learning and literacy, vol. 7. Lawrence Erlbaum Associates; 2007. Available at. http://ncsall.net/fileadmin/resources/ann_rev/rall_v7_ch6.pdf. Accessed August 1, 2019.

12. US Department of Health and Human Services. An issue brief from the U.S. Department of Health and Human Services. America's Health Literacy: why we need accessible health information. 2008. Available at: https://health.gov/communication/literacy/issuebrief. Accessed August 1, 2019.

13. Haymond S. What everyone should know about lab tests: they aren't always correct and they aren't always useful. Scientific American 2016. Available at: https://blogs.scientificamerican.com/guestblog/what-everyone-should-know-about-lab-tests/. Accessed August 1, 2019.

14. Lippi G, Favaloro EJ, Plebani M. Direct-to-consumer testing: more risks than opportunities. Int J Clin Pract 2011;65:1221–9.

15. Keselman A, Slaughter L, Smith CA, et al. Towards consumer-friendly PHRs: patients' experience with reviewing their health records. AMIA Annu Symp Proc 2007;399–403.

16. Zarcadoolas C, Vaughon WL, Czaja SJ, et al. Consumers' perceptions of patient-accessible electronic medical records. J Med Internet Res 2013;15:e168.

17. Tolan NV. Direct-to-consumer testing: a new paradigm for point-of-care testing. Point of Care 2017;16:108–11.

18. Safeer RS, Keenan J. Health literacy: the gap between physicians and patients. Am Fam Physician 2005;72:463–8.

19. Berkman ND, Dewalt DA, Pignone MP, et al. Literacy and health outcomes. (AHRQ Publication No. 04-E007-2). Rockville, MD: Agency for Healthcare Research and Quality; 2004.

20. Direct Access Testing (DAT) and the Clinical Laboratory Improvement Amendments (CLIA) regulations. Center for medicare and medicade services. Available at: https://www.cms.gov/Regulations-and-Guidance/Legislation/CLIA/Downloads/directaccesstesting.pdf. Accessed August 1, 2019.

21. Direct Access Testing. Position paper: consumer access to laboratory testing and information. McLean, VA: American Society for Clinical Laboratory Science; 2012.

Available at: https://www.ascls.org/position-papers/179-direct-access-testing/155-direct-access-testing. Accessed August 1, 2019.

22. Baudhuin LM. The FDA and 23andMe: violating the First Amendment or protecting the rights of consumers? Clin Chem 2014;60:835–7.
23. Rockwell KL. Direct-to-consumer medical testing in the era of value-based care. JAMA 2017;317:2485–6.
24. Zafar HM, Bugos EK, Langlotz CP, et al. "Chasing a Ghost": factors that influence primary care physicians to follow up on incidental imaging findings. Radiology 2016;281:567–73.
25. van der Wouden CH, Carere DA, Maitland-van der Zee AH, et al. Consumer perceptions of interactions with primary care providers after direct-to-consumer personal genomic testing. Ann Intern Med 2016;164:513–22.
26. Bloss CS, Wineinger NE, Darst BF, et al. Impact of direct-to-consumer genomic testing at long term follow-up. J Med Genet 2013;50:393–400.
27. At FTC's PrivacyCon. Concerns about the monetization of consumer health data. Portland, ME: MobiHealthNews, HIMSS Media; 2016. Available at: https://www.mobihealthnews.com/content/ftcs-privacycon-concerns-about-monetization-consumer-health-data. Accessed August 1, 2019.
28. Regalado A. More than 26 million people have taken an at-home ancestry test. MIT Technology Rev 2019. Available at: https://www.technologyreview.com/s/612880/more-than-26-million-people-have-taken-an-at-home-ancestry-test/. Accessed August 1, 2019.
29. Scutti S. What the golden state killer case means for your genetic privacy. New York, NY: CNN Health, Warner Media Group; 2018. Available at: https://www.cnn.com/2018/04/27/health/golden-state-killer-genetic-privacy/index.html. Accessed August 1, 2019.
30. Adam S, Friedman JM. Individual DNA samples and health information sold by 23andMe. Genet Med 2016;18:305–6.
31. Keshavan M. 20 key players in the direct-to-consumer lab testing market. MedCity News; 2016. Available at: https://medcitynews.com/2016/01/20-key-players-in-the-direct-to-consumer-lab-testing-market/. Accessed August 1, 2019.
32. General Accountability Office. Nutrigenetic testing: tests purchased from four web sites mislead consumers. GAO-06-977T. 2006. Available at: https://www.gao.gov/products/GAO-10-847T. Accessed August 1, 2019.
33. General Accountability Office. Direct-to-consumer genetic tests: misleading test results are further complicated by deceptive marketing and other questionable practices. GAO-10-847T. 2010. Available at: https://www.gao.gov/products/GAO-10-847T. Accessed August 1, 2019.
34. Neighmond. U.S. Justice Department charges 35 people in fraudulent genetic testing scheme. Shots Health News from NPR. 2019. Available at: https://www.npr.org/sections/health-shots/2019/09/27/765230011/u-s-justice-department-charges-35-people-in-fraudulent-genetic-testing-scheme. Accessed October 17, 2019.
35. Gronowski AM, Haymond S, Master SR. Improving direct-to-consumer medical testing. JAMA 2017;318:1613.
36. Haymond S, Grenache D, Holmes D, et al. Three ways DTC testing can better serve consumers' needs – we can improve at-home lab tests. USNews World Rep 2016. Available at: http://www.usnews.com/opinion/articles/2016-06-28/3-ways-to-improve-direct-to-consumerhealth-tests-like-theranos-and-23andme. Accessed August 1, 2019.

Direct-to-Consumer Tests on the Market Today

Identifying Valuable Tests from Those with Limited Utility

Timothy Scott Isbell, PhD, DABCC

KEYWORDS

- Direct-to-consumer testing • Direct access testing • Value • Clinical utility
- Analytical validity

KEY POINTS

- Value is subjective, being defined by different perspectives. Consumers identify entertainment, altruism, health knowledge, and financial value in direct-to-consumer (DTC) testing.
- Health care professionals have expressed concern regarding selection, interpretation, clinical utility, and analytical validity of DTC testing.
- DTC testing is here to stay and predicted to grow, and laboratory medicine professionals are uniquely qualified to educate the public about the limitations of DTC testing and study DTC testing–related clinical outcomes.

DIRECT-TO-CONSUMER TESTING DEFINED

The U.S Food and Drug Administration (FDA) defines direct-to-consumer (DTC) tests as in vitro diagnostic assays that are marketed directly to consumers without the involvement of a health care provider.[1] The ability to purchase laboratory testing without a physician's order varies from state to state, with most states allowing for some form of what is often referred to as direct access testing (DAT). In states where DAT is permissible, patients simply order and pay for tests online and then present to an authorized draw station for sample collection. Patient reports are typically accessed through a secured Web site. Physician consults are sometimes offered for an additional price.

The largest proportion of DTC testing by volume is genetic, allowing consumers to probe their own genome for information about disease risk, inheritable traits, ancestry, and familial relationships. In 2018, the DTC genetic testing market was valued at 831.5 million USD and is expected to grow to 2.5 billion USD by 2025,

Department of Pathology, Division of Clinical Pathology, Saint Louis University School of Medicine, St. Louis, MO, USA
E-mail address: scott.isbell@health.slu.edu

Clin Lab Med 40 (2020) 13–23
https://doi.org/10.1016/j.cll.2019.11.008
0272-2712/20/© 2019 Elsevier Inc. All rights reserved.

labmed.theclinics.com

per a recent market analysis performed by Global Market Insights.[2] DTC tests are heavily marketed to consumers through all outlets: television, radio, print, and social media. As reported by *MIT Technology Review* in 2016, Ancestry and 23andMe invested substantial amounts in marketing their product, 109 million and 23 million USD, respectively.[3]

However, not all DTC tests are genetic. An entire nongenetic market exists, allowing individuals to, for example, purchase panels of laboratory tests, have their microbiome analyzed, and measure "toxins" in their blood and urine. **Table 1** lists specific examples of DTC genetic products versus nongenetic DTC tests.

In addition to QuestDirect and WellnessFx listed (see **Table 1**), there are many other Web sites that offer the ability for individuals to order their own laboratory tests, including but not limited to the following:

- Walk-in-Lab
- HealthOneLabs
- Personalabs
- Request A Test
- DirectLabs

These sites allow individuals to shop for a variety of single-analyte or multianalyte panels of laboratory tests.

Consumer interest in DTC testing is driven in part by a desire to have more control over one's health. More than ever, individuals are engaged and actively searching for information about their health online and via wearable devices that provide continuous streams of biometric data, from number of steps (distance) taken in a day to heart rate, sleep patterns, and now cardiac rhythm.

Position or policy statements from professional laboratory medicine–related organizations, including the American Association for Clinical Chemistry, the American Society of Clinical Pathology, and the American Association for Clinical Laboratory Science, indicate general support for access to DTC testing but with the following stipulations[4–6]:

- Testing should be performed in a Clinical Laboratory Improvement Amendments (CLIA)-certified laboratory.
- Consumers of DTC should be provided access to expert consultation to assist with ordering and interpretation.
- Consumers should work with qualified health care professionals in making decisions affecting their own health, including sharing results of DTC testing.

The American College of Medical Genetics articulated the following positions in 2015[7]:

- The clinical testing laboratory must be accredited by CLIA.
- A genetics expert, such as a certified medical geneticist or genetic counselor, should be available to help the consumer determine, for example, whether a genetic test should be performed and how to interpret these results considering personal and family history.
- The consumer should be informed regarding what the test can and cannot say about their health.
- The consumer should be apprised of the potential for receiving results that can neither confirm nor rule out the possibility of disease or unexpected results that are unrelated to the specific reason for testing as well as the implications of genetic testing results for family members.

- The scientific evidence base describing the validity and utility of a genetic test should be clearly stated.
- Privacy concerns must be addressed.

The ability to order and view one's laboratory data is similarly on the increase. Haymond and colleagues[8] in a 2016 *US News and World Report* article noted, "direct-to-consumer labs meet patients' desire for on-demand services with mobile-friendly user interfaces enabling prompt return of results at relatively low out-of-pocket expense."

Table 1
Examples of genetic versus nongenetic direct-to-consumer tests

Genetic Based DTC Testing Product	Company	Claim[a]	Price, USD[a]
Health + ancestry (includes health predispositions, ancestry, wellness, carrier status, traits)	23andMe	Health predispositions: Learn how your genetics can influence your chances of developing certain health conditions	149
Mayo Clinic GeneGuide	Helix	A genetic testing experience that helps you understand how genetics can affect your health. Get personalized insights, interactive tools, and education that help you explore the health information in your DNA, carrier screening, disease risk, family health history, and more	149
Diet Fit	DNAfit	Discover how your genetics affect the way you metabolize carbohydrates & fats, to build your personal plate. Discover how your DNA can signal a raised need for certain vitamins and nutrients. Discover recipes, advice, and shopping lists that are built for you and only you. Based on your genetic results, along with your goals and preferences	89
Paternity testing	LabCorp. Inc	Paternity testing provides scientific evidence of whether a man can be a child's biological father. Paternity is determined by comparing the child's DNA with the DNA profile of the alleged father	210 (at home testing) 525 (legal)
AncestryDNA	Ancestry	This service combines advanced DNA science with the world's largest online family history resource to predict your genetic ethnicity and help you find new family connections	99
Infidelity DNA test	EasyDNA	Cheating is no longer about guess work. The infidelity DNA test is ideal to help provide a good indication of whether cheating has taken place. Clients can send in a variety of different samples, which have roused their suspicions. An infidelity test can be carried out using a range of DNA samples, including nail clippings and hairs	299

Non-Genetic-Based DTC Testing Product	Company	Claim[a]	Price, USD[a]
Men's Health Profile	QuestDirect	This screening for men includes a prostate health test and everything in the Basic Health Profile, for a comprehensive look at overall health. It can help identify a wide range of possible health conditions so you can take informed action toward your health goals	199
Explorer	uBiome	uBiome Explorer kits give you access to state-of-the-art tools to learn more about your microbiome. Explore your gut microbiome at a single time point and see how you compare with other Explorer users	89
Performance	WellnessFX	Having the complete picture of your health works to eliminate the guesswork and gives you data you can then take meaningful action on. Testing includes total cholesterol, HDL, LDL, triglycerides, Lp(a) ApoB, TSH, glucose, HbA1c, DHEA, free testosterone, testosterone, estradiol, SHBG, 25-hydroxy-VitD, calcium, electrolytes, bicarbonate, hs-CRP, BUN/creatinine, AST, ALT, total bilirubin, albumin, total protein, cortisol, IGF-1, insulin, ferritin, total iron binding capacity, folate, vitamin B12, RBC magnesium	497

[a] Extracted from company Web site, accessed October 7, 2019.

Many concerns have been raised regarding the value of DTC testing. Complicating this debate is the difficulty of defining "value." Value can be defined differently depending on the perspective taken, a point highlighted nicely by Dr. David Grenache[9] in a 2017 *Clinical Chemistry* article, wherein he states, "as with any service or product, the consumer makes the determination regarding value." One can argue, however, that different stakeholders possess differing views on the value of DTC testing. Herein, the author attempts to define value relative to multiple perspectives.

VALUE FROM THE PERSPECTIVE OF THE CONSUMER

Per the *Merriam-Webster Dictionary*, value can be defined as the noun meaning: (1) the monetary worth of something; (2) a fair return or equivalent in goods, services, or money for something exchanged; (3) relative worth, utility, or importance. The word "utility" is often used as a synonym for value in discussions about DTC testing. The ever-expanding market of DTC testing is in part evidence that the consumer finds value in DTC testing given their willingness to pay for these services. Types of value from the perspective of the consumer may be categorized in the following manner.

Entertainment Value

A subset of DTC genetic testing is primarily intended to provide entertainment to the end-user. For example, DTC genetic testing is available that informs consumers about a variety of inheritable traits from the ability to match musical pitch and asparagus odor detection, to earlobe type, aversion to cilantro, and earwax type. DTC genetic testing that informs individuals about their ancestry is very popular among amateur and professional genealogists. Per a recent article in *MIT Reviews Technology*, an estimated 26 million people have taken an in-home ancestry test, representing roughly 8% of the US population, and that number is expected to grow to around 100 million within the next 2 years.[10] DTC genetic testing, which informs the user of inheritable traits and ancestral information, is considered low risk because there is no predictable health-related action that can be taken from such information.

Health Knowledge Value

In a systematic review of the literature on consumer perspectives regarding DTC genetic testing, Goldsmith and colleagues[11] identified the following reasons individuals pursued DTC genetic testing:

- Learn about individual genetic risk
- Lifestyle modification if increased risk for disease is identified
- Increase control over their health
- Stimulate family discussion over health
- Take personal responsibility for future health
- Convey risk to children
- Assist primary care physician with health monitoring

Companies such as 23andMe now have FDA clearance to market DTC genetic testing. The DTC tests with market authorization following an evaluation by the FDA for accuracy, reliability, and consumer comprehension are summarized in **Table 2**, modified from a public notice provided by the FDA.[1]

DTC testing offers an opportunity to address a need expressed by individuals with chronic disease. In a survey of individuals with at least 1 chronic disease, conducted between December 2016 and January 2017 by West Corporation, 70% of respondents indicated they would like more resources on how to manage their disease, and 91% indicated they need help managing their disease at home between doctor's visits. Ninety-four percent of survey respondents indicated that the use of 2-way biometric monitoring technology would be somewhat to very helpful.[12] The best example of at-home monitoring of chronic disease is self-monitoring of blood glucose in the setting of diabetes mellitus, a standard of care per the American Diabetes Association for patients with insulin-dependent diabetes.[13]

Opportunities for at home management of chronic disease using DTC testing include the following:

- Measurement of whole blood capillary glucose for correction of hyperglycemia and detection of hypoglycemia
- Measurement of hemoglobin A1C to monitor long-term glycemic control
- Measurement of urine ketones to screen for ketosis in patients with diabetes
- Measurement of urine albumin-to-creatinine ratio in the setting of chronic kidney disease
- Measurement of plasma lipids to assist with goal-directed therapy (lifestyle modifications and/or medications)
- Measurement of tumor biomarkers to monitor for cancer reoccurrence

Measurement of these analytes as prescribed by a physician has been shown to improve outcomes as part of chronic disease management. Except for capillary whole

Table 2
Food and Drug Administration–cleared direct-to-consumer tests

Trade Name	Intended Use
23andMe PGS Carrier Screening Test for Bloom Syndrome	Detection of the BLMAsh variant in the BLM gene from saliva. This test can be used to determine carrier status for Bloom syndrome in adults of reproductive age, but cannot determine if a person has 2 copies of the BLMAsh variant
23andMe PGS Genetic Health Risk Test	The 23andMe Personal Genome Service (PGS) Test uses qualitative genotyping to detect the following clinically relevant variants in genomic DNA isolated from human saliva: • Hereditary thrombophilia (factor V Leiden variant in the F5 gene, and the prothrombin G20210A variant in the F2 gene) • Alpha-1 antitrypsin deficiency (PI*Z and PI*S variants in the SERPINA1 gene) • Late-onset Alzheimer disease (ε4 variant in the APOE gene) • Parkinson disease (G2019S variant in the LRRK2 gene and the N370S variant in the GBA gene) • Gaucher disease type 1 (N370S, 84GG, and V394L variants in the GBA gene) • Factor XI deficiency (F283L, E117X, IVS14+1G > A in the F11 gene) • Celiac disease (HLA-DQ2.5 haplotype) • Glucose-6-phosphate-dehydrogenase deficiency (Val68Met variant in the G6PD gene) • Hereditary hemochromatosis (C282Y and H63D variants in the HFE gene) • Early-onset primary dystonia (DYT1/TOR1A-related) (deltaE302/303 variant in the DYT1 gene).
23andMe PGS Genetic Health Risk Report for BRCA1/BRCA2 (selected variants)	The 23andMe PGS Genetic Health Risk Report for BRCA1/BRCA2 (selected variants) is indicated for reporting of the 185delAG and 5382insC variants in the BRCA1 gene and the 6174delT variant in the BRCA2 gene
23andME PGS Pharmacogenetic Reports	The 23andMe PGS Pharmacogenetic Reports are indicated for reporting of the following variants: *Gene* *Variant(s)* CYP2C19 *2, *3, *17 CYP2C9 *2, *3, *5, *6, rs7089580 CYP3A5 *3 UGT1A1 *6, *28 DPYD *2A, rs67376798 TPMT *2, *3C SLCO1B1 *5 CYP2D6 *2, *3, *4, *5, *6, *7, *8, *9, *10, *11, *15, *17, *20, *29, *35, *40, *41

Adapted from U.S. Food & Drug Administration. Direct-to-consumer tests. Available at: https://www.fda.gov/medical-devices/vitro-diagnostics/direct-consumer-tests.

blood glucose, the serial measurement of these analytes as directed by consumers has yet to be shown to improve outcomes.

In the acute setting, DTC testing for sexually transmitted infections (STIs) has in theory the opportunity to help lower disease burden by improving access to testing.

Recent data from the Centers for Disease Control and Prevention demonstrate, relative to 2014, increases in chlamydia, gonorrhea, and syphilis infections by 19%, 63%, and 71%, respectively, with an alarming 185% increase in congenital syphilis.[14] DTC testing for STIs is readily available online, requiring blood collected at home (via capillary stick) to be mailed to a clinical laboratory for analysis and reporting. At home testing for human immunodeficiency virus (HIV) using the OraQuick testing system was approved by the FDA in 2012. OraQuick does not require sending a sample to a laboratory but rather works by detecting antibodies to HIV-1 and -2 in oral fluid specimens. With a sensitivity of 91.7% and a specificity of 99.9%, per the manufacturer's package insert, concerns have been raised about potential false negatives, especially during the window period. A failure to fully appreciate these testing limitations could lead to continued disease transmission if in fact the individual was HIV positive and failed detection by the home test. Moreover, with self-testing, results are not guaranteed to be communicated to public health authorities. Proponents of self-testing for HIV within the home argue increased access especially in communities that would otherwise not get tested because of cultural constraints. In the end, access to testing is but 1 part of the equation: linkage to care and management with antiretroviral therapy are required to reduce the transmission of HIV.

Altruistic Value

DTC genetic testing companies offer the ability for consumers of their products to participate in research by agreeing to share their genetic data and other data collected as part of electronic surveys. Participation in biomedical research appeals to many individuals' sense of altruism and the desire to be part of something bigger than them. In fact, the 23andMe Web site informs viewers that, "our genetic research gives everyday people the opportunity to make a difference by participating in a new kind of research—online, from anywhere."

Per the company's Web site, "the 23andMe database is a rich resource, with genotypic and phenotypic information from more than 5 million of our customers, 80 percent of whom consent to participate in 23andMe research. By consenting to participate, our customers agree to make their de-identified genetic data available for study in aggregate and take part in online research under a protocol approved by an external institutional review board (IRB)." 23andMe partners with academic institutions, industry, and nonprofits to share the data they collected in the hopes of making scientific and medical advances. These partnerships have led to the publication of 140 papers in respected peer-reviewed journals, such as *Nature Genetics*, *Science*, and *New England Journal of Medicine*.

Financial Value

Within the United States, the costs of clinical laboratory testing provided as part of routine medical care can be very expensive even for individuals with health insurance. For individuals with no health insurance, laboratory testing can quickly get into the thousands of dollars. Determining the price for laboratory tests within the health care system is challenging for consumers given the nonstandardized charges and variable pricing negotiated between health insurance companies and health care facilities. In contrast, DTC or DAT clinical laboratory testing provides market-driven, transparent pricing that allows for individuals to shop around for the best price usually at prices far cheaper than what is available through health care providers. Health Tests Direct advertises "order blood tests online! Save 50–81% here. Skip the Doctor...the exam room...the wait time...all that inconvenience!" **Table 3** provides average test prices for routine laboratory tests.

Table 3
Average calculated cost of routine testing based on pricing quoted online from 3 different direct access testing providers: health test direct, QuestDirect, and DirectLabs

Test	Average Price in USD (Standard Deviation)
Complete blood count	27.60 (2.4)
Urinalysis	38.24 (1.3)
Complete metabolic panel	37.33 (10.4)
Hemoglobin A1c	37.19 (3.1)

VALUE FROM THE PERSPECTIVE OF THE HEALTH CARE PROVIDER

To the health care provider, the value of DTC testing is focused more on the associated clinical utility. In a perspective piece, Delaney and Christman[15] make the argument that value in medical genetics can be thought of as clinical utility, with clinical utility demonstrated if the information gained from the DTC genetic test leads to action, provides a definitive diagnosis, or serves to supplement family history.

DTC pharmacogenomic testing is emerging as perhaps an area of DTC genetic testing with the most potential to generate actionable information, especially if the information helps to optimize medications and dosage to avoid adverse drug events. However, concerns exist around applicability of screening for Asian, African American, and Hispanic populations, detection of copy number variants, and self-management of medications without physician or pharmacist input.

Findings from the Impact of Personal Genomics study indicated 54 (5.6%) individuals reported changing a medication they were taking, or starting a new medication, because of their DTC-pharmacogenomic testing (PGT) results with 16.7% not consulting with a health care provider regarding the change.[16] Individuals should be advised to consult a licensed health care provider before adjusting drug dosage to avoid potential adverse events associated with overdosage and underdosage of medications.

Health care professionals' concerns around DTC testing mainly center on the following:

- Data interpretation
- Analytical validity
- Clinical utility
- Lack of outcomes data

In their 2015 position statement, the American College of Medical Genetics expressed concern regarding the interpretation of DTC genetic testing and recommends that consumers be aware of the limitations of such tests given that DTC genetic tests do not provide a definitive answer regarding disease development but rather provide information about risk or probability of developing disease. Moreover, they recommend that results be interpreted by a board-certified genetics professional.[7] A similar concern has been raised regarding the interpretation of nongenetic DAT. Skeptics of DAT question the ability of the individuals to appropriately interpret the details of clinical laboratory results, whereby misinterpretation could lead to a false reassurance or unnecessary worry and additional testing. In addition, there is concern regarding the self-ordering of clinical laboratory tests to "screen for disease" given the lack of appreciation regarding the increased probability of false positive results when tests are ordered in individuals with a low pretest probability for the disease or condition. Follow-up on false positive results from DTC testing can lead to unnecessary testing and costs.

Many of the DTC tests available online to consumers contradict evidence-based medical practice guidelines. A study by Lovett and colleagues[17] found that out of 127 different tests only 4 (3%) had evidence to support screening in the general population and only 19 (15%) could be supported for screening in a targeted group. The remaining tests evaluated had recommendations against testing in select populations, insufficient evidence for screening, or no guidance given. Collectively, the investigators concluded that "virtually all identified medical tests advertised and offered direct-to-consumer are not recommended for use in screening by evidence based guidelines."

For health care professionals, the analytical validity of DTC tests is a primary concern. Analytical validity of DTC genetic testing can be defined by analytical sensitivity and specificity whereby analytical sensitivity is defined as how often a test is positive when the genetic variant of interest is present in the tested sample, and the analytical specificity is defined as how often a test result is negative when the tested sample does not contain the genetic variant of interest.[18] A recent study by Tandy-Connor and colleagues[19] "indicated that 40% of variants in a variety of genes reported in DTC raw data were false positives" when compared with clinical confirmatory testing. This study highlights the need to scrutinize the analytical validity of DTC genetic testing and consider confirmatory testing in a clinical diagnostic genetics laboratory. Per the American Society of Human Genetics, "companies offering DTC genetic testing should disclose the sensitivity, specificity and predictive value of the test, and the populations for the information is known, in a readily understandable and accessible fashion."[20]

There are few data examining outcomes associated with DTC testing. Most studies have focused on examining behavioral changes in individuals purchasing DTC testing. A study by Bloss and colleagues[21] examined the long-term (1-year follow-up) impact of DTC testing and found no negative psychological risks for individuals participating in DTC genetic testing and found that one-third of individuals surveyed shared their DTC results with their physician. A similar study by the same group found increased physician utilization and no adverse changes in psychological health in a cohort of individuals submitting to DTC pharmacogenomic testing.[22] In a follow-up study of individuals receiving DTC genetic testing results indicating increased cancer risk, no significant changes were noted in diet, exercise, advanced care planning, or cancer screening behaviors at 6 months.[23] Additional longitudinal studies are needed to determine the association between DTC testing and morbidity/mortality.

Taken together, the concerns regarding selection, interpretation, performance, and the paucity of clinical outcomes data related to DTC testing should serve as a call to action for health care professionals, especially those with training in laboratory medicine. Laboratory medicine professionals are uniquely qualified to study and generate best practice data for optimal use of DTC testing, which could include recommending for or against DTC testing depending on outcomes data. Regardless of eventual recommendations that should follow outcomes-based studies of DTC testing, laboratory medicine professionals have an immediate duty to educate the public about the limitations of DTC testing and provide direction regarding evidence-based practice guidelines.

RISK MITIGATION

As highlighted earlier, DTC testing is associated with the risk of false negative and false positive results, which can lead to a false sense of assurance that all is well on the part of the consumer or can lead to unnecessary psychological stress and additional testing and costs, respectively. Mitigation of this risk requires education and consultation. Consumers need to be informed about the relative risk of self-directed testing; the limitations of an assay should be explained in understandable terms, and access to experts, preferably health care professionals, should be made available to answer questions and provide direction. Results of DTC testing should be shared with the health care professional as supplements to standards of care. Consumers should avoid taking care into their own hands and should discuss changes in lifestyle and any prescribed medications. Laboratory medicine professionals should be knowledgeable about the scope of DTC testing and should advocate that testing adhere to the same standards applied in the hospital and other clinical settings. Moreover, laboratory medicine professionals should work together to educate the public about the value and limitations of laboratory testing.

SUMMARY

In this information age, demand for health-related information will continue to grow as more and more individuals take ownership of their health. DTC testing is here and predicted to expand. Value is subjective, but evidence-based clinical outcomes are not. It must recognized that consumers find value in these DTC tests, while at the same time research should be continued to evaluate the impact of DTC testing on health and provide best practice recommendations.

DISCLOSURE

The author has nothing to disclose.

REFERENCES

1. Direct-to-consumer tests US Food and Drug Administration. Available at: https://www.fda.gov/medical-devices/vitro-diagnostics/direct-consumer-tests. Accessed October 3, 2019.
2. Ugalmugale S. Direct-to-consumer genetic testing market. Selbyville, DE: Global market insights; 2019:.
3. Regaldo A. 2017 was the year consumer DNA testing blew up. MIT Technology Review; 2018.
4. Direct access testing (policy number 01-02).. American Society for Clinical Pathology: Chicago, IL Available at: https://www.ascp.org/content/docs/default-source/policy-statements/ascp-pdft-pp-direct-access-testing.pdf?sfvrsn=2. Accessed October 16, 2019.
5. Direct-to-consumer laboratory testing. Washington, DC: American Association for Clinical Chemistry; 2015. Available at: https://www.aacc.org/health-and-science-policy/advocacy/position-statements/2015/direct-to-consumer-laboratory-testing. Accessed October 7, 2019.
6. Consumer access to laboratory testing and information. McLean, VA: American Society for Clinical Laboratory Science; 2012. Available at: https://www.ascls.org/position-papers/179-direct-access-testing/155-direct-access-testing. Accessed October 7, 2019.
7. ACMG Board of Directors. Direct-to-consumer genetic testing: a revised position statement of the American College of Medical Genetics and Genomics. Genet Med 2016;18(2):207–8.
8. Haymond S, Grenache D, and Master S. We Can Improve At-Home Lab Tests: Here are 3 ways direct-to-consumer testing can better serve consumers' health

needs. US News and World Report. June 28, 2016. Available at: https://www.usnews.com/opinion/articles/2016-06-28/3-ways-to-improve-direct-to-consumer-health-tests-like-theranos-and-23andme. Accessed October 16, 2019.

9. Li M, Diamandis EP, Grenache D, et al. Direct-to-consumer testing. Clin Chem 2017;63(3):635–41.
10. Regaldo A. More than 26 million people have taken an at-home ancestry test. Cambridge, MA: MIT Technology Review; 2019.
11. Goldsmith L, Jackson L, O'Connor A, et al. Direct-to-consumer genomic testing: systematic review of the literature on user perspectives. Eur J Hum Genet 2012; 20(8):811–6.
12. Corporation W. Strengthening chronic care–patient engagement strategies for better management of chronic conditions 2017. Available at: https://www.televox.com/downloads/west_chronic_disease_report.pdf. Accessed October 16, 2019.
13. Diabetes technology: standards of medical care in diabetes. American Diabetes Association (ADA)2019. Diabetes Care 2019;42(Supplement 1):S71–80.
14. Centers for Disease, C. Sexually transmitted disease surveillance 2018. U.S. Centers for Disease Control and Prevention. Available at: https://www.cdc.gov/std/stats18/toc.htm. Accessed October 14, 2019.
15. Delaney SK, Christman MF. Direct-to-consumer genetic testing: perspectives on its value in healthcare. Clin Pharmacol Ther 2016;99(2):146–8.
16. Carere DA, VanderWeele TJ, Vassy JL, et al. Prescription medication changes following direct-to-consumer personal genomic testing: findings from the Impact of Personal Genomics (PGen) Study. Genet Med 2017;19(5):537–45.
17. Lovett KM, Mackey TK, Liang BA. Evaluating the evidence: direct-to-consumer screening tests advertised online. J Med Screen 2012;19(3):141–53.
18. National Research Council (US) and Institute of Medicine (US) Roundtable on Translating Genomic-Based Research for Health. Direct-To-Consumer Genetic Testing: Summary of a Workshop. Washington (DC): National Academies Press (US); 2010. Scientific Foundations for Direct-to-Consumer Genetic Testing. Available at: https://www.ncbi.nlm.nih.gov/books/NBK209647/.
19. Tandy-Connor S, Guiltinan J, Krempely K, et al. False-positive results released by direct-to-consumer genetic tests highlight the importance of clinical confirmation testing for appropriate patient care. Genet Med 2018;20(12):1515–21.
20. Hudson K, Javitt G, Burke W, et al. ASHG statement on direct-to-consumer genetic testing in the United States. Am J Hum Genet 2007;81(3):635–7.
21. Bloss CS, Wineinger NE, Darst BF, et al. Impact of direct-to-consumer genomic testing at long term follow-up. J Med Genet 2013;50(6):393–400.
22. Bloss CS, Schork NJ, Topol EJ. Direct-to-consumer pharmacogenomic testing is associated with increased physician utilisation. J Med Genet 2014;51(2):83–9.
23. Gray SW, Gollust SE, Carere DA, et al. Personal genomic testing for cancer risk: results from the impact of personal genomics study. J Clin Oncol 2016;35(6): 636–44.

Challenges with At-home and Mail-in Direct-to-Consumer Testing
Preanalytical Error, Reporting Results, and Result Interpretation

Kornelia D. Galior, PhD, DABCC[a], Nikola A. Baumann, PhD, DABCC[b],*

KEYWORDS

- DTC testing • Total testing process • Preanalytics • Postanalytics

KEY POINTS

- Direct-to-consumer (DTC) testing empowers consumers by providing direct access to laboratory testing and results.
- Consumers should be aware of the challenges and limitations of DTC testing.
- DTC testing should not be treated as a substitute for a routine health assessment.
- Follow-up of potentially actionable DTC test results requires involvement of health care providers and confirmatory testing in a clinical laboratory.

INTRODUCTION

The brain-to-brain turn-around time loop for laboratory testing, proposed by Lundberg in 1981,[1] conceptualized a framework for the total testing process required to produce laboratory results. The total testing process includes 3 phases: preanalytical, analytical, and postanalytical. The preanalytical phase encompasses the steps from when the test is ordered by the health care provider and the specimen is collected from the patient until the specimen is ready to analyze. The analytical phase occurs during sample analysis. The last phase, termed the postanalytical phase, consists of all the steps that occur after the analysis is complete, including laboratory result reporting and result interpretation. Compartmentalization of laboratory testing into preanalytical, analytical, and postanalytical phases has been the foundation for quality improvement in the clinical laboratory over the past 40 years.

[a] Department of Pathology and Laboratory Medicine, University of Wisconsin School of Medicine and Public Health, 600 Highland Ave Madison, WI 53792, USA; [b] Department of Laboratory Medicine and Pathology, Mayo Clinic, 200 First St SW, Hilton 3-70, Rochester, MN 55905, USA
* Corresponding author.
E-mail address: Baumann.Nikola@mayo.edu

Clin Lab Med 40 (2020) 25–36
https://doi.org/10.1016/j.cll.2019.11.006   labmed.theclinics.com
0272-2712/20/© 2019 Elsevier Inc. All rights reserved.

The process was aptly termed the "brain-to-brain loop" because it began and ended with decisions made by the clinician; that is, the clinician's brain. The beginning of the loop was the health care provider deciding which laboratory test was appropriate for her or his patient and the loop closed with the physician interpreting the information from the laboratory and making clinical decisions for the patient. Interestingly, the patient was a rather passive "specimen donor" in the laboratory total testing process.

The emergence of direct-to-consumer (DTC) laboratory testing challenges the conceptual framework of Lundberg's[1] brain-to-brain loop. The most dramatic change is that the brain-to-brain loop begins and ends with the consumer: the patient determines what laboratory tests to order and receives the laboratory test results and any interpretive information (**Fig. 1**). The extent of a clinician's involvement is at the discretion of the patient.

DTC laboratory testing can provide individuals with the empowerment of requesting available testing based on their personal desire for knowledge and having direct access to their own data. However, as with clinical laboratory results, there are many factors that can affect the accuracy of DTC testing results at multiple steps in the total testing process. As a result, concerns have been raised about the appropriate use, accuracy, and the quality of DTC test results.[2] The subsequent sections discuss the total testing process for both clinical laboratories and DTC testing, specifically addressing the unique challenges associated with DTC testing.

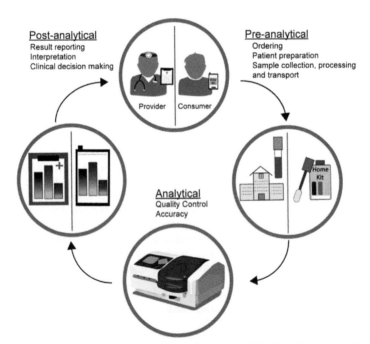

Post-analytical
Result reporting
Interpretation
Clinical decision making

Pre-analytical
Ordering
Patient preparation
Sample collection, processing
and transport

Provider | Consumer

Analytical
Quality Control
Accuracy

Fig. 1. The total testing process includes preanalytical, analytical, and postanalytical phases, with each phase encompassing numerous steps. The major differences between conventional laboratory testing and DTC testing are that the consumer is responsible for the steps in the preanalytical phase and most of the postanalytical phase, including interpretation of results and deciding whether follow-up is required. In conventional laboratory testing, the total testing process is managed within the health care system.

OVERVIEW OF DIRECT-TO-CONSUMER TESTING

DTC tests are laboratory tests that are marketed directly to consumers without the involvement of a health care provider.[3] DTC tests span the spectrum of laboratory tests from over-the-counter (OTC) pregnancy tests and home glucose testing, to highly complex genetic testing. Some DTC tests are marketed to consumers as screening tests for diseases including cancer and cardiac disease.[4,5] Other companies market "health tests" that range from analyzing blood biomarkers (vitamins, lipids, cardiovascular markers, thyroid and reproductive hormones) to screening for parasites, heavy metals, and toxins. Available DTC genetic tests offer to provide an array of information including ancestry, risks of developing certain conditions, carrier status for autosomal recessive diseases, and information about nondisease phenotypic traits.

BENEFITS AND CHALLENGES OF DIRECT-TO-CONSUMER TESTING

Having access to long-standing DTC tests, such as human immunodeficiency virus tests, pregnancy tests, glucometers, and even home thermometers, has improved the diagnosis and monitoring of disease and empowered consumers to take control of specific aspects of their health care. In some cases, the availability and privacy of DTC tests may reduce the anxiety associated with visiting a physician and as a result may allow earlier knowledge and intervention. The success stories of DTC testing reside with testing that is easy for the consumer/patient to understand, that is, a positive pregnancy test indicates pregnancy; or where patient/consumer education has been made a priority, that is, glucose monitoring in the diabetic patient population. In these situations, there is benefit to DTC home testing.

There is currently sparse scientific information that shows effectiveness of DTC testing in disease prevention. However, a positive consequence of DTC testing would be the identification of increased risk in unsuspecting patients or results that would allow a patient to take preventive action, make lifestyle changes, or seek earlier clinical intervention and follow-up within the health care system. An unintended consequence of DTC testing is the scenario in which additional testing and follow-up in the health care setting may be unnecessary, causing increased burden and cost to the system and increased anxiety and cost to the patient. A false-negative DTC test result, interpreted by a consumer, could conversely falsely reassure a patient who might otherwise seek health care within the conventional health care system.

DIRECT-TO-CONSUMER GENETIC TESTING

In the United States, the DTC genetic testing arena has changed dramatically over the past decade. Although the evolving regulatory and ethical considerations are outside of the scope of this article, they are discussed elsewhere within this issue (See L.M. Peterson and J.A. Lefferts's article, "Lessons Learned from Direct to Consumer Genetic Testing," and the A.M. Grownoski and M.M. Budelier's article, "The Ethics of Direct to Consumer Testing"). The Food and Drug Administration (FDA) currently regulates DTC genetic testing and restricts DTC genetic testing companies from offering products that function as diagnostic tests. In 2015, the first genetic carrier screen received FDA device approval, and in 2017, DTC genetic health risk tests became available. A broad spectrum of DTC genetic testing is now readily available, including carrier testing for diseases such as cystic fibrosis and hemochromatosis; pharmacogenomic testing; testing for predisposition to complex diseases such as hereditary cancers, cardiovascular disease, and depression; whole exome or genome sequencing; and ancestry determination.[6]

Companies offering DTC genetic testing are primarily accessed by consumers via Internet sites. Consumers can order specimen collection kits online and kits are subsequently shipped to the consumer with instructions for specimen collection. The consumer collects his or her own specimen, usually saliva or a buccal swab, and then mails the specimen to the company. The specimen is analyzed and results are obtained and posted on a secure Web site that is accessible only to the purchaser and the company. Consumers are often asked to provide consent that the genetic data obtained may be used by the company for further studies.

Genetic test interpretation in the traditional health care setting often involves genetic counselors who are trained to help patients understand complex genetic test results and possible implications for patients and family members. For medical conditions, DTC genetic testing is currently available to assess risk of developing certain diseases; however, concepts such as "increased risk" or "low risk" are not easily translatable to binary interpretation (ie, positive or negative for given disease).

NONGENETIC DIRECT-TO-CONSUMER TESTING

Nongenetic DTC testing has a variety models, including OTC home test kits or drop-in clinics or pharmacies, where blood tests are offered directly to consumers without requiring a physician requisition. The test menu available to consumers encompasses much of the clinical laboratory test menu. Frequently tests are offered as packages to assess "wellness" or "metabolic health" and include a variety of hormones, vitamins, trace metals, or other tests. The steps in this model of testing closely mimic the total testing process of conventional clinical laboratories. Because of this similarity, the challenges and opportunities for error are comparable. However, under the veil of non-diagnostic, wellness, testing outside of a Clinical Laboratory Improvement Amendments (CLIA)-regulated laboratory, the requirements for quality assurance are reduced, or altogether nonexistent.

TOTAL TESTING PROCESS: THE PREANALYTICAL PHASE

The preanalytical phase is the first phase in the laboratory testing process. This phase includes many steps starting with the physician ordering the appropriate test, ensuring proper patient preparation and identification, to correctly collecting, transporting, and processing the specimen before analysis. In the laboratory total testing process, the preanalytical phase tends to be the most vulnerable to errors because it occurs almost entirely external to the clinical laboratory. Ordering the wrong test(s), improper labeling of specimens or lack of positive patient identification, incorrect patient preparation (eg, not fasting), or difficult phlebotomy are some examples of preanalytical errors that can affect certain laboratory test results. Delays in transportation and specimen processing, exposure of specimens to inappropriate temperature and light during transportation, or improper storage conditions are also significant contributors to errors in the preanalytical phase.

To minimize errors, trained health care professionals perform most, if not all, of the preanalytical phase of laboratory testing. In addition, health care facilities and laboratories must have written policies and procedures for correctly identifying, collecting, and handling specimens throughout the preanalytical phase, including processes for handling deviations from the standard protocol.

The preanalytical phase is dramatically different for DTC testing. The process begins when the consumer, not physician, determines the need for a laboratory test. The consumer now plays the role of ordering physician by determining which test to order and must ensure that the specimen is properly collected. Depending on the test, consumers then either label, package, and transport the specimen to the testing entity or perform the test themselves according to the manufacturer's instructions.

Patients Order the Direct-To-Consumer Tests

In contrast to the traditional clinical testing system, the DTC testing system starts with a consumer, not a physician, placing an order for the test (**Table 1**). For OTC, home-based DTC testing, the kit includes both a specimen collection and testing device (ie, urine pregnancy kits). For other DTC testing, a kit including a saliva, buccal swab, or blood collection device, or urine container is sent directly to the consumer's home where the consumer collects the specimen. For DTC laboratory testing offered at clinics and pharmacies, blood collection is performed by employees of the company. The required specimen is then mailed to the company or contracted laboratory for analysis. Results are generally available via an easily accessible Web-based portal or laboratory results are sent directly to the patient. Depending on the results, the company may release the results with interpretations and/or recommendations regarding diet, supplements, exercise, and lifestyle.

Initiatives to order the right test on the right patient at the right time have been a focus of quality improvement initiatives and best practices in laboratory medicine. Strategies such as clinical decision support at order entry and laboratory formularies that restrict ordering of laboratory tests that are nonessential or have limited utility are widely used in health care. DTC testing enables patients to have essentially unre-stricted access to an array of laboratory testing that may or may not be appropriate

Table 1
Differences between direct-to-consumer (DTC) testing and conventional clinical laboratory testing

Step in Total Testing Process	Conventional Health Care System with Clinical Laboratory Testing	Direct-to-Consumer Testing
Laboratory test ordering	Physician orders tests after clinical assessment of patient	Consumer self-orders tests based on demand and availability
Patient preparation	Patient provided instructions by health care provider	Consumer follows instructions on kit or from DTC company
Specimen collection, processing, and transport	Trained health care professionals collect and process according to documented procedures	Consumer follows manufacturer instructions
Analytical quality control	Regulatory requirements for quality control and laboratory oversight	Variable, testing may or may not have regulatory oversight
Result reporting and interpretation	Health care provider responsible for reviewing results and discussing with patient Patient may have direct access to results	Consumer receives report and interprets
Follow-up and clinical decision making	Health care provider determines appropriate action and discusses options with patient	Consumer is responsible for follow-up

for their personal medical situation. Although this availability of options may initially be appealing to the consumer, the risk of unintended consequences is important and is discussed later in this article.

Patient Preparation

Patient-specific factors, such as ambulation, body posture before collection, exercise, stress, and diurnal variation, are common preanalytical factors that may affect laboratory results. These variables are often communicated to the patients and accounted for by health care professionals; however, in case of DTC testing, the consumer must be made aware of and understand these factors. For example, ambulation before specimen collection can impact the concentration of total proteins, lipids, and other protein-bound substances. Concentration of hormones, such as cortisol, growth hormone, and other hormones, varies throughout the day, so collection needs to be accurately timed. Recent ingestion of food greatly impacts concentration of triglycerides, glucose, and other substances, so length of fasting before specimen collection is an important variable.

Sample Collection

Regardless of the specimen required, proper sample collection is an important step for obtaining accurate results. For DTC genetic tests using saliva or buccal swab collections, consumers must follow kit instructions and adhere to special instructions, such as not eating, drinking, chewing gum, or brushing teeth for defined times before sampling. DTC blood tests may use capillary blood obtained via fingerstick collections, which are also susceptible to collection errors. The type of lancet; selection of puncture site on the finger; proper cleansing, disinfection, and drying; and avoiding applying too much pressure around the puncture site are all important for obtaining a quality specimen. Incorrect collection by applying excessive pressure to the finger will cause interstitial fluid to dilute the blood sample and effectively dilute the sample leading to falsely low analyte concentrations. For DTC tests requiring venous blood collection, correct venipuncture technique also is critical. Venipuncture errors include prolonged tourniquet application time, incorrect order of collection for tubes containing additives (order of draw) (eg, sodium citrate for coagulation, K-EDTA for hematology), underfilling of collection tubes containing additives, contamination, and hemolysis. Hemolysis, or lysis of red blood cells, is a rather commonly encountered preanalytical issue and can have a clinically significant impact on many laboratory tests because of release of intracellular analytes into the serum or analytical interference with colorimetric methods due to the red pigment.

Sample Identification

Proper patient identification and specimen identification are considered a priority for patient safety in the health care setting. Verbal confirmation of at least 2 patient identifiers (ie, name and date of birth or medical record number) combined with barcoded labels and/or radiofrequency identification tracking are used to confirm specimen identification throughout the total testing process. In DTC testing, the consumer is the patient, so the risk of accidental misidentification by way of switching a sample with another individual is low. However, intentional misidentification of specimens can occur if someone were to collect a sample from another individual and send it under his or her own identification. One of the early DTC genetic testing companies celebrated their launch by having Spit Parties where attendees danced, drank, and submitted DNA samples for sequencing.[7] That era of DTC genetic testing has ended; however, it remains unclear how such companies confirm patient and specimen identity throughout the testing process or how they would detect a misidentified specimen. Conventional clinical laboratories have regulatory requirements and processes for positive specimen identification and patient/specimen identification is confirmed throughout the total testing process.

Transportation and Storage

Following the proper technique and procedures for specimen collection, transportation, and processing are critical for obtaining accurate laboratory results. Even with clearly defined processes, rejecting specimens that were delayed in transit or transported under incorrect conditions is not uncommon in the clinical laboratory. Within health care systems, there is attention to details such as transporting specimens at the correct temperature and ensuring that analysis occurs within a defined time frame and under conditions in which the analyte is known to be stable. In clinical laboratories, appropriate specimen storage conditions that ensure analyte stability are either obtained from the manufacturer's instructions for use for FDA-cleared tests or validated independently by the laboratory. Criteria for acceptable storage and time frames are part of the analytical standard operating procedures in the clinical laboratory. Samples are electronically tracked so that important time stamps, such as time of collection and time of reporting, are monitored. Delays in transportation or specimen processing, exposure of specimens to inappropriate temperature during transportation, or improper storage conditions can be significant contributors to laboratory errors and erroneous results. For DTC testing, samples are collected and shipped, if necessary, by the consumer following instructions provided by the DTC company. The impact of incorrect collection, transport conditions, or storage on test results has not been reported for DTC testing. Although there is a void of information, one can assume that improper handling of specimens does occur and may negatively impact the accuracy of test results.

TOTAL TESTING PROCESS: THE ANALYTICAL PHASE

The analytical phase includes all the processes involved with the analysis of the specimen. Traditionally, this phase is considered the least prone to error because it occurs entirely within the clinical laboratory and is closely monitored by quality control processes and procedures.

Using analytical methods with known and validated accuracy and precision can also help to minimize analytical errors. It is important to note that analytical errors do occur and laboratory quality control processes must be robust and designed to detect analytical errors in real-time. This is particularly important in high-volume, high-throughput laboratories where an analytical error can quickly impact numerous test results if not detected. With DTC testing, there have been concerns about the accuracy of the test results that are not performed by the CLIA- or College of American Pathologists (CAP)-accredited laboratories.[8,9]

OTHER CONTRIBUTORS TO ANALYTICAL QUALITY: SAMPLE INTEGRITY AND INTERFERENCES

Although sample integrity may be compromised during the preanalytical phase of testing by variables such as patient preparation or collection technique, the assessment of sample integrity most often occurs during the analytical phase. Analytical quality assurance tools in the clinical laboratory include the use of automated serum indices that semiquantitatively assess the extent of hemolysis, icterus, or lipemia present in the sample and assist in determining whether the sample is suitable for analysis. For example, analytes that are highly concentrated within red blood cells will be released when hemolysis occurs. Analytes such as potassium, aspartate aminotransferase, and lactate dehydrogenase will not be accurate in hemolyzed samples. Lipemia can impact indirect ion selective electrode measurements as well as some spectrophotometric measurements. It is critical that laboratories define thresholds for acceptable serum indices and mitigation strategies for handling compromised samples.

Interference with analytical methods also can occur in patients with certain medical conditions, those taking certain medications or vitamins, and individuals with specific antibodies that can cross-react with the test reagent components. Although it is impossible to predict or detect every possible interference, quality laboratory results require diligence on the part of the laboratory and communication with the physician who is interpreting the results. In many cases, interferences can be detected and mitigated by the laboratory; however, in some cases they are identified only because the test result is inconsistent with the patient's clinical presentation and history. One example of an interference being difficult to detect is the interference caused by OTC hair, skin, and nail supplements containing high concentrations of biotin. At high enough concentrations, biotin interferes with some immunoassays because it binds to the components of the reagents used to measure molecules such as thyroid hormones and cardiac biomarkers, among others. Although laboratorians and clinicians are aware of this type of interference and how to troubleshoot suspected interference, consumers may not be aware of the risk.

DTC laboratories should adhere to the same good laboratory practices as clinical laboratories; however, without accreditation or regulatory oversight, it is difficult to assess whether this occurs. In addition, the laboratorian/clinician dialogue does not exist in the DTC model and consumers may not have enough experience or knowledge to be aware of interferences or results that are inconsistent with each other or with the clinical context in which they were measured.

TOTAL TESTING PROCESS: THE POSTANALYTICAL PHASE

The postanalytical phase includes all of the steps after the analytical result is obtained and includes laboratory result reporting, result interpretation, and appropriate clinical decision making, follow-up, and action.

Result Reporting

Traditionally, the clinical laboratory delivered patient laboratory results via reports intended to be read, interpreted, and communicated to patients by their health care provider. The laboratory provided interpretive information but there was an assumption that concepts such as clinical sensitivity, clinical specificity, reference intervals, therapeutic indices, risk, and medical decision points were understood by the physician who had ordered the laboratory tests. The physician would be familiar with the patient's clinical history, symptoms, and physical examination, and be able to interpret the laboratory results in conjunction with clinical findings. Importantly, a clinician also would be able to recognize when laboratory results were not consistent with clinical findings and when to suspect false-positive or false-negative test results. All of this information would be communicated to the patient by his or her health care provider.

The advent of patient portals where patients directly receive their laboratory results via secure Web-based apps or private health care accounts is a paradigm shift. It is commonplace for patients to receive their laboratory results in real-time and often before physicians review the results themselves and in turn, communicate with the patients. However, even with patient portals, the physician is still responsible for ordering the test, reviewing the patient's results, and providing feedback and necessary follow-up on abnormal results.

DTC testing shifts the paradigm even further because the consumer is usually the sole recipient of the laboratory results and the consumer is left to interpret the results and decide how to proceed.

In simplistic terms, laboratory results assist in differentiating health versus disease. However, many laboratory findings are not simply interpreted as positive or negative and even those that are, have intrinsic sensitivity, specificity, and positive and negative predictive value that must be considered in the context of the patient's presentation of symptoms and/or clinical history.

Laboratory Result Interpretation

Reference intervals

Many laboratory results are reported in the context of a reference interval; that is, the expected range of values observed in a healthy reference population. On laboratory result reports, values outside of that range are usually flagged as abnormal. Typically, if a reference interval is defined as the central 95th percentile of a reference population, then one would expect that 5% of the reference population would have values outside of the reference interval. Hence, one would also expect that 5% of healthy patients will have laboratory values outside of the central 95th percentile reference interval.[10] As the number of laboratory tests ordered increases, the probability of a test result falling outside of the reference interval by chance alone is 1 minus 0.95^n when n tests are performed. For example, if 14 tests are ordered on a completely healthy individual, the probability of 1 result falling outside of the reference interval just due to random variation is greater than 50%. Although the information contained in laboratory reports varies, descriptions of reference intervals and criteria for flagging results are usually not described.

Many consumers will use the Internet to search for information about their laboratory results. Lab Tests Online (LTO) is an online resource where patients, their family members, and health care professionals can learn more about the tests used to screen for, diagnose, and manage disease.[11] LTO is an important tool but it does not provide reference intervals with test interpretation information because of the lack of harmonization between laboratories and potential to mislead users. Campbell and colleagues[11] reported that, according to focus group data, the general public was surprised and even shocked to find that reference intervals are subject to interlaboratory variation and not standardized.

Health literacy and direct-to-consumer genetic testing

Health literacy is the ability of consumers of health care to read, understand, and act on health information. Interpretation of laboratory results requires not only reading comprehension but also numeracy, the ability to read and interpret numerical information.[11] It is recommended that patient education materials and health information sites should have content written at a fourth to sixth grade level. Translating this recommendation to the DTC era would suggest that laboratories providing DTC services should be providing laboratory reports, including the numeric results, interpretation, and limitations, in a format that is easily understood at a sixth grade reading level.

With increased oversight by the FDA of DTC genetic testing, the FDA confirmed that the DTC company 23andMe had submitted extensive analytical validation data for their carrier screen for the hereditary Bloom Syndrome, as well as evidence establishing that members of the public were capable of correctly interpreting the test report at a 90% comprehension level.[7] These data were not published, but the idea that user comprehension of test results should be part of DTC test validation is an excellent step in the right direction. Unfortunately, it is not currently a requirement.

Consumer Follow-up to Direct-to-Consumer Test Results

On receiving the DTC test results, a consumer interprets the results and is left to decide appropriate next steps. If laboratory reports are comprehensive and clear, the risk of inappropriate action is low. However, a lack of understanding and heavy reliance on DTC test results may lead to self-misdiagnosis, anxiety, or taking inappropriate actions.

Perhaps the best case scenario is that the consumer will follow-up with their health care provider. However, one could question whether this leads to more direct expense for the patient and cost to the health care system.

SHOULD HEALTH CARE PROVIDERS USE DIRECT-TO-CONSUMER TEST RESULTS?

Consumers may give authorization to share the DTC laboratory test results with their health care provider or they may share the results directly. If the results of the DTC testing suggest increased risk for disease or abnormal results, the patient will likely need to go to his or her health care provider for appropriate follow-up. In most cases, follow-up will include confirmatory diagnostic tests and clinical assessment under the oversight of the health care provider.

Should health care providers make clinical decisions based on DTC laboratory testing? At this time, the answer is no, based on the rather limited data available. There have been concerns about the accuracy of DTC test results.[8] Theranos was a notable player in the DTC testing market touting availability of routine laboratory tests (ie, chemistry, immunoassay, and hematologic testing) using small blood volumes from finger sticks instead of needle-collected venipuncture. One study compared blood tests obtained from a finger prick performed at a retail outlet (Theranos) and 2 major clinical testing services that required standard venipuncture draws (Quest and Lab-Corp). The investigators found that Theranos flagged test results outside of their normal range 1.6 times more often than the other testing services, and 68% of the laboratory measurements showed significant interlaboratory variability.[9] It is worth mentioning that Theranos subsequently dissolved in 2018 after the company faced serious legal problems and received sanctions from the Centers for Medicare and Medicaid Services, including revocation of its CLIA certificate. The cofounder, Elizabeth Holmes, was charged with "massive fraud" by the US Securities and Exchange Commission.

Genetic test results are inherently complex and often require interpretive reports in addition to genetic counselor involvement when delivering results to patients. Some DTC genetic testing companies will provide raw genotyping data to the consumer if requested. The raw data may include clinically significant or actionable variants occurring in genes. One study reviewed the outcome of 49 requests for clinical confirmation of DTC results and found that 40% of the variants in genes reported in DTC raw data were false positives.[12] The same investigators identified variants that were classified by the DTC company as "increased risk" in the DTC raw data but were classified as "benign" by several clinical laboratories. In light of the FDA authorizing, with special controls, DTC genetic testing for assessing hereditary breast cancer risk (BRCA), Reed and Edelman[6] published the following recommendations for clinicians presented with such results: (1) before using DTC test results (positive or negative) to make clinical decisions, results need to be confirmed in a clinical laboratory on a new sample; (2) negative results on DTC testing are not definitive, additional testing may be needed if there is clinical indication of higher risk; and (3) positive results on DTC testing can help identify individuals who did not know they were at risk.

These studies highlight the risk of performing laboratory testing outside of the conventional clinical laboratory.

SUMMARY

The growing market for DTC testing provides an opportunity to promote awareness of laboratory testing among the general public. Consumers have become more knowledgeable about their health and want to take a proactive role in their overall health management and care, including greater access to laboratory tests and interpretation of laboratory information. However, the expansion of DTC testing to include accessibility to more laboratory tests and high complexity tests brings the following challenges that need to be addressed:

- DTC testing should adhere to the same quality requirements as conventional laboratory testing during the total testing process.
- Consensus on which DTC tests provide value to consumers and guidance for appropriate consumer utilization (as well as cautions about inappropriate utilization).
- DTC test result reports should be clear, include limitations of testing, and suggest appropriate follow-up.
- Understanding how DTC test results are used and whether DTC is causing unnecessary follow-up with health care providers or providing important diagnostic information is needed.[13]

With increasing experience in the era of DTC testing, consumer risks and benefits will continue to emerge and evolve.

REFERENCES

1. Lundberg GD. Acting on significant laboratory results. JAMA 1981;245(17):1762–3.
2. Rockwell KL. Direct-to-consumer medical testing in the era of value-based care. JAMA 2017;317(24):2485–6.
3. Schwartz LM, Woloshin S. Medical marketing in the United States, 1997-2016. JAMA 2019;321(1):80–96.
4. Lovett KM, Liang BA. Direct-to-consumer cardiac screening and suspect risk evaluation. JAMA 2011;305(24):2567–8.
5. Lovett KM, Mackey TK, Liang BA. Evaluating the evidence: direct-to-consumer screening tests advertised online. J Med Screen 2012;19(3):141–53.
6. Reed EK, Edelman EA. Direct-to-consumer genetic testing for breast cancer risk. J Am Assoc Nurse Pract 2018;30(10):548–50.
7. Allyse MA, Robinson DH, Ferber MJ, et al. Direct-to-consumer testing 2.0: emerging models of direct-to-consumer genetic testing. Mayo Clin Proc 2018;93(1):113–20.
8. Lippi G, Favaloro EJ, Plebani M. Direct-to-consumer testing: more risks than opportunities. Int J Clin Pract 2011;65(12):1221–9.
9. Kidd BA, Hoffman G, Zimmerman N, et al. Evaluation of direct-to-consumer low-volume lab tests in healthy adults. J Clin Invest 2016;126(7):2773.
10. Katayev A, Balciza C, Seccombe DW. Establishing reference intervals for clinical laboratory test results: is there a better way? Am J Clin Pathol 2010;133(2):180–6.

11. Campbell B, Linzer G, Dufour DR. Lab tests online and consumer understanding of laboratory testing. Clin Chim Acta 2014;432:162–5.
12. Tandy-Connor S, Guiltinan J, Krempely K, et al. False-positive results released by direct-to-consumer genetic tests highlight the importance of clinical confirmation testing for appropriate patient care. Genet Med 2018;20(12):1515–21.
13. Gronowski AM, Haymond S, Master SR. Improving direct-to-consumer medical testing. JAMA 2017;318(16):1613.

Self-Ordering Laboratory Testing

Limitations When a Physician Is not Part of the Model

Daniel T. Holmes, MD[a,b],*

KEYWORDS

- Direct-to-consumer testing • Genetics • Genomics • FDA
- US Food and Drug Administration • CLIA-waived • Point of care

KEY POINTS

- The direct-to-consumer (DTC) paradigm disrupts the traditional laboratorian/clinician/patient triad.
- The risks of DTC testing are often invisible to patients, and even to their clinicians, because of general unfamiliarity with the discipline of pathology and laboratory medicine.
- Patients are unprepared to evaluate laboratory diagnostics as consumer products making them vulnerable to exploitation.
- DTC testing flies in the face of efforts within traditional health care sectors to use evidence-based approaches and diagnostic stewardship programs to prevent waste.

BACKGROUND

Direct-to-consumer (DTC) diagnostic testing is not a new concept. The first over-the-counter glucose monitors for the management of diabetes mellitus became available in the early 1980s[1] and the first at-home urine pregnancy kits were marketed in the United States in 1978, touted in advertisements as "the private little revolution."[2] Subsequently, devices for ovulation,[3] international normalized ratio (INR),[4] urine drugs of abuse, human immunodeficiency virus,[5] and hepatitis C testing[6] all have been successfully marketed. Nowadays, these are more or less considered regular consumer products like toothpaste and acetaminophen sold ubiquitously from pharmacies. Despite the fact that INR devices have suffered from analytical performance issues

[a] Department of Pathology and Laboratory Medicine, St. Paul's Hospital, 1081 Burrard Street, Vancouver, British Columbia V6Z 1Y6, Canada; [b] Department of Pathology and Laboratory Medicine, University of British Columbia, G105-2211 Wesbrook Mall, Vancouver, British Columbia V6T 2B5, Canada
* Department of Pathology and Laboratory Medicine, St. Paul's Hospital, 1081 Burrard Street, Vancouver, British Columbia V6Z 1Y6, Canada.
E-mail address: dtholmes@mail.ubc.ca

Clin Lab Med 40 (2020) 37–49
https://doi.org/10.1016/j.cll.2019.11.002
0272-2712/20/© 2019 Elsevier Inc. All rights reserved.
labmed.theclinics.com

leading to device[7] and test-strip recalls by the Food and Drug Administration (FDA),[8] it can only be expected that the menu of DTC tests available over the counter will continue to grow. Point-of-care devices sold from pharmacies represent only 1 category of DTC testing.

Wherever there are buyers, sellers will avail themselves and, in time, non–Clinical Laboratory Improvement Amendments–waived moderate or high complexity biochemical tests have been marketed on a DTC basis from accredited diagnostic laboratories. Although numbers may be shifting, 1 study observed that 34 American states permit this form of DTC testing, either because the law is silent on the matter or limited access to DTC testing is explicitly permitted.[9] Another less regulated form of testing, usually ordered by practitioners of naturopathy, is available from nonaccredited facilities promoting testing of questionable medical and scientific merit. This article makes no distinction between DTC testing obtained by a patient without any request from a health practitioner and testing ordered by a naturopath. The rationale behind this decision is that in the paradigm of naturopathy, patients are acting as consumers of services and functionally speaking can direct the services (laboratory or otherwise) they wish to purchase. It is acknowledged that some might dispute this assertion. Finally, and perhaps most conspicuously, testing for a wide array of conditions and genetic susceptibilities has been available since approximately 2003[10] and has been the subject of continuous and evolving FDA scrutiny.[11]

This review discusses how the DTC paradigm disrupts the traditional laboratorian/clinician/patient triad, highlighting the risks to patient well-being that ensue. These risks usually are invisible to patients, as medical consumers, and sometimes even to clinicians because of their unfamiliarity with the discipline of pathology and laboratory medicine. Using Lyme disease testing as an example paradigm, I review how patients are unprepared to evaluate laboratory diagnostics as a consumer product and how this has made them vulnerable to exploitation. I also discuss the manner in which DTC testing flies in the face of concerted efforts within traditional health care sectors to apply principles of evidence-based medicine and diagnostic stewardship to prevent overutilization and waste.

LABORATORY TESTING IS DIFFERENT FROM CONSUMER PRODUCTS

Almost all consumer products can be effectively evaluated by the purchaser through product use, and defective wares can be identified and returned for refund. Sellers who abuse their customer base by deliberately distributing defective goods are subject to swift retribution through online consumer forums and social media. Restaurants can be evaluated by the quality of the food; retailers by the quality of the clothing ,electronics or cookware; service industries by their hours of operation, courteousness, and efficacy.

Laboratory testing is different. Only the preanalytical phase (How long did I wait? How polite was the staff? and How painless was the sample collection?) and the postanalytical phase (How quickly did the report arrive? How readable is the report? and Is the report aesthetically pleasing?) can be evaluated by the consumer. The most important part of the testing, however, namely, How accurate is the result? remains entirely opaque. In the DTC laboratory testing paradigm, consumers have no way to kick the tires on tests themselves, except perhaps if they reveal a clear diagnosis that can be confirmed and managed or cured. This likely explains why the infamous DTC laboratory Theranos was able to continue garnering venture capital funding and mislead even savvy clinicians with a great deal of expertise in laboratory medicine[12] while internally the Theranos laboratory showed shocking noncompliance with legally mandated quality-control procedures.[13]

Physician's Role in Laboratory Quality Assessment

Physicians have served as both diagnosticians and caregivers throughout the history of Western medicine. In this role, they act as stewards of the available diagnostic resources (including of their own time and clinical skills), interpreters of the findings, deliverers of therapeutic intervention, protectors of patients' private health information, and their advocate to other health care workers. Through experience and practice, a physician learns when a physical finding or diagnostic result is clinically significant, when it should be assigned low significance, and even when it should be ignored. When a laboratory result does not make clinical sense, it is the physician's role to question the validity of the result, repeat the testing, or perform follow-up testing as appropriate. It is also the physician's role to assess the quality of the overall diagnostic testing process (to whatever extent possible) and either provide feedback to the laboratory or, alternatively, direct the patient to a different laboratory facility as required. Physicians have the necessary training and experience to assess diagnostic services on behalf of their patients—not unlike their role in serving as advocates for other health care resources, such as social services and nursing. The clinician's role is mirrored within the laboratory by the clinical pathologist and the other medical professionals (clinical chemists, clinical microbiologists, and clinical geneticists), who seek to provide the physician with the best possible diagnostic information, interpret or assist in the interpretation of testing, and steward the available resources to optimize the care delivered to all patients. The laboratory physicians and scientific professionals in turn hold diagnostic companies accountable for the quality of clinical diagnostic equipment and consumable reagents.

This means that there is an appropriate tension at every stage of laboratory medicine care where medical caregivers in the laboratory act to represent patient needs to diagnostic companies whereas clinicians represent patient needs to laboratory medicine professionals, and patients represent their own needs to their clinician. This loop of dialectics prevents any one group's interests from being overrepresented and maintains a patient's well-being as the primary aim of all involved parties, defending the patient against several potential threats.

The Wrong Test from a Good Laboratory

For the most part, any group of related laboratory tests that might be ordered, in particular routine tests (eg, complete blood cell count and electrolytes), do not result in a diagnostic smoking gun. They are part of a mosaic formed from the clinical history, physical examination, laboratory testing, and medical imaging, which are assembled by a clinician to formulate diagnosis and treatment plan. Although exceptionally motivated patients may be able to research the meaning of an abnormal result, they are incapable of objectivity, even if the patients themselves are physicians, which is why in some jurisdictions, physicians are forbidden by licensing bodies[14] or strongly discouraged by professional associations[15] from ordering tests or prescriptions on themselves or their relatives except in extenuating circumstances. Even if the laboratory of choice produces excellent quality results, patients have no experience by which to select or interpret the tests. Neither do they have the objectivity to interpret the tests and order downstream tests in an unbiased and impartial manner. A typical diagnostic testing formulary has a few hundred to even thousands of selections, none of which has any meaning to the general public except those whose interpretation is part of common life experience, such as pregnancy and HIV testing.

Disparate Laboratory Quality

Not all laboratories perform to the same standards, as evidenced by disparate performance on external quality-assurance assessments. This is well known within laboratory medicine circles but less appreciated by clinicians. Most clinicians, however, do generally have the perspective to recognize when a laboratory result or an entire laboratory should be subjected to skepticism. Patients, on the other hand (and even some clinicians), assume that diagnostic tests always are accurate and have no appreciation for patient factors (eg, time of day, dietary, and medication effects), preanalytical factors, random analytical error, bias, and interferences. For this reason, abnormal results are overinterpreted, as has been shown by programs offering patients access to their results through Internet portals.[16,17] It is known that testing leads to more testing[18] and the obvious concern is that patients, when acting as their own diagnosticians, will order tests in the wrong clinical context (ie, tests for conditions with low pretest likelihood), receive ambiguous or confusing diagnostic reports, and either pursue further testing through their primary care physician or, worse, purchase more testing entirely on their own.

Laboratories Offering Non–evidence-based Testing

In addition to laboratories offering traditional evidence-based diagnostic menus, there are an increasing number of DTC companies offering testing services targeted to naturopaths and wellness/integrative medicine clinics. Although these facilities may use some of the same analytical techniques as traditional diagnostic laboratories, they frequently offer testing demonstrating marginal or even dubious scientific support. For example, they may offer hormone panels in salivary matrix—without disclosing that this stretches their immunoassays into concentration domains, where analytical performance is abysmal. Alternatively, they may measure long lists of hormones for which the clinical meaning is completely unestablished. From the perspective of patients, the public presence of a glossy website, the convenience of an easily collected sample, and the measurement of a very long list of analytes impart perceived value, as does an aesthetically pleasing report. This gives patients a sense that they are receiving better (newer and cutting-edge) service, whereas the reality is that they may be receiving no value except the greater possibility of an abnormal report.

UNWARRANTED INVESTIGATIONS: STATISTICAL CONSIDERATIONS

Even if it is idealistically assumed that the reference intervals in a laboratory are perfectly set to flag reports outside the central 90%, 95% or 99% of results collected from healthy subjects, the probability of at least 1 abnormal result grows with the number of tests performed, as shown in **Fig. 1**.

This means that in a complete blood cell count panel, typically of 20 parameters, using central 95% reference intervals, there is an approximately 65% chance of at least 1 test flagging as abnormal in the absence of any clinical abnormality. Naturally, a patient cannot be expected to understand the nuance of type I (false-positive or false-discovery) errors[19] as they apply to diagnostic testing. As discussed previously, the detection of abnormal test results leads to further downstream diagnostic testing and therapeutic intervention even when testing is directed by a physician or medical team. Even in settings that seem medically appropriate, such as inherited thrombophilia testing in the context of prior arterial stroke, there is a risk of harm associated with the diagnostic findings and the associated interventions.[20,21] Ordering that is not driven by appropriate clinical motivations, such as by medicolegal defensiveness, worsens the overall outcome of patient care.[22]

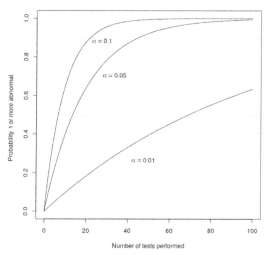

Fig. 1. Probability of at least 1 flagged test for reference intervals defined by the central 90% ($\alpha = 0.1$), 95% ($\alpha = 0.05$) , and 99% ($\alpha = 0.01$) of a healthy population.

An important related concept to false discovery is that of Bayes theorem, which describes the mathematical relationship between the pretest and post-test odds of disease given a positive test result. Specifically, it illustrates that if the test is performed in the wrong clinical context, one in which a patient has a low pretest probability, the post-test odds of disease will be low no matter the quality of the diagnostic testing process. Considering a test for which the diagnostic specificity (rate of negativity in health) and sensitivity (rate of positivity in disease) are established,[23] the post-test odds of disease after a positive test ($odds_{post}$) can be found by multiplying the likelihood ratio of a positive test result (LR^+) by the pretest probability ($odds_{pre}$):

$$odds_{post} = LR^+ \times odds_{pre}$$

where,

$$LR^+ = \frac{sensitivity}{1 - specificity}$$

A mathematical consequence is that positive test results in the setting of low disease prevalence are likely to be false positives because positive predictive value (PPV) correspondingly diminishes according to the following formula:

$$PPV = \frac{sensitivity \times prevalence}{sensitivity \times prevalence + (1 - specificity) \times (1 - prevalence)}$$

As the prevalence of a disease in the test populations gets close to 0, this equation can then be approximated by the following:

$$PPV_{low\ prev} \approx \frac{sensitivity \times prevalence}{1 - specificity} = LR^+ \times prevalence$$

which clearly illustrates that the PPV is directly proportional to the prevalence in the low prevalence limit. A likelihood ratio of greater than 10 is considered good for a diagnostic test but if the prevalence of a disease is only 0.5%, then the PPV for a test with

$LR^+ = 10$ is only 5%. Because this concept is unappreciated by most medical professionals, it can scarcely be expected that patients will understand it. Therefore, if a patient selects diagnostics tests inappropriate to the symptoms (which is probable when symptoms are vague and inevitable for wellness testing), nearly all positives will be false positives, rendering the downstream clinical diagnostic follow-up/testing needless and wasteful.

DOWNSTREAM TESTING

In the DTC paradigm, patients are the initiators of downstream investigations and can pursue further diagnostic testing on their own without the help of a physician caregiver. Conceivably, patients may even alter their treatment (eg, change or stop taking their prescriptions) based on inaccurate or misinterpreted laboratory results. This undermines the appropriate feedback that both physician and patient receive as part of their relationship with one another and the laboratory, short-circuiting the so-called brain-to-brain loop that describes the diagnostic process[24,25] and allowing the patient to struggle, expending emotional and financial resource without experience, expertise, or guidance on the complex topic of human pathophysiology.

Even when they pursue the help of a physician, caregivers often are placed in the awkward position of following-up on testing that have been ordered on appropriate clinical grounds, and they may feel pressured to undertake therapy or investigations that have risks associated with them.

Case Example: Lyme Disease Testing

Lyme disease testing represents a good case study for the effects of the DTC testing market because the testing has been available for more than 2 decades, the impacts have been studied, and the quality of the DTC tests have been characterized.

Lyme disease is caused by an infection from the spirochete *Borrelia burgdorferi* and is transmitted by the bite of the *Ixodes scapularis* and *Ixodes pacificus* tick species. It is a multisystem illness affecting the skin, muskuloskeletal, nervous, and cardiovascular systems. Acute Lyme disease has some fairly specific clinical manifestations, notably erythema migrans, which classically presents as a target-like annular rash at the site of the tick bite, typically appearing within 1 week to 2 weeks of the initial exposure. The rash is accompanied by pronounced constitutional symptoms: fever, malaise, myalgia, arthralgia, and lymphadenopathy.[26] A clinical history of travel walking, hiking, or camping in endemic areas, with or without recollection of a bite, together with clinical and laboratory findings permits an early diagnosis and treatment with appropriate antibiotic therapy with amoxicillin, doxycycline, or cefuroxime.

If an infection is not identified in its early stages, a patient may go on to develop hematogenous spread of the spirochete and multiple erythema migrans lesions similar in appearance to the primary lesion. Fever, malaise, fatigue, myalgias, and arthralgias persist and subsequently neurologic, rheumatological, and cardiac findings may develop, for example, facial nerve palsy, oligoarticular arthritis (particularly of the knee), and atrioventricular block.[27] Arthritis may persist after antibiotic therapy and often has an autoimmune component.

The most pertinent entity for the present discussion is so-called chronic Lyme disease. This term is slightly confusing because it encompasses several conditions, namely, late untreated Lyme disease and post–Lyme disease syndrome,[26,28] which is characterized by nonspecific findings, such as headache, fatigue, sleep disorders, and a long list of other vague symptomatology outlined in a dedicated guidance document.[29] The clinical definition of chronic Lyme disease has such broad symptomatology so as to easily be mistaken for several rheumatological and neurologic conditions, including osteoarthritis, rheumatoid arthritis, degenerative spinal diseases, peripheral neuropathies, multiple sclerosis, and amyotrophic lateral sclerosis.[30]

Given the prevalence of nonspecific fatigue and musculoskeletal symptoms in the middle-aged population[31] and the growing popularity of naturopathic clinics, so-called wellness practitioners and integrative health clinics,[32] the diagnostic possibility of chronic Lyme disease is attractive, whether rational or not, because it represents an opportunity for patients to vindicate their experiences, providing them an explanation for their symptoms and hope for a cure. Accordingly, whether by pure or tainted motives, an industry of Lyme disease serologic testing has sprung up in both the United States and Canada. These laboratories may have false-positive rates greater than 50% in healthy individuals,[33,34] indicating either that the antibodies used are nonspecific or that the threshold for declaring a positive test is too low, resulting in poor clinical specificity. In 1 study using chronic fatigue syndrome and systemic lupus erythematosus as controls, no subjects with previously diagnosed Lyme disease by privately obtained serologic testing were confirmed to have Lyme disease by a reference laboratory using multitier staged testing.[35] Notwithstanding specific advice against use of a single serologic western blot by the US Centers for Disease Control[36,37] and clear guidance on optimal diagnostic strategy,[38] the industry around Lyme disease testing shows no evidence of curtailment[39] even in the pediatric population.[40]

As discussed previously, consumers are unable to distinguish clinical diagnostic testing from salesmanship on the part of private testing companies and may view the failure of clinical diagnostic laboratories to detect Lyme disease (or other illnesses) as evidence of their inadequacy, unaware of the false-positive results they have received. Primed by a long list of nonspecific clinical findings associated with chronic Lyme disease,[29] patients easily fall victim to their own confirmation bias. At this stage, it is distinctly advantageous to the DTC companies to reinforce this bias by undermining clinical diagnostic and clinical reference laboratories for using what they allege is "inferior" testing of inadequate sensitivity—a strategy commonly used. Well-intentioned though may be, this notion is echoed by Lyme disease patient advocacy groups who do not appear to understand the trade-offs between sensitivity and specificity in diagnostic testing.

There eventually may develop a conspiratorial sentiment on the part of the patient-consumer that traditional diagnostic and reference laboratories are collectively misguided or deliberately ill-intentioned. By way of example from outside the context of Lyme disease per se, but squarely inside the paradigm of DTC testing, prominent venture capitalist and Theranos financial backer Tim Draper repeatedly and publicly accused Theranos detractors of being backed by "Big Pharma", belying either naivety for the distinction between the diagnostic and pharmaceutical industries or intent to deliberately misdirect the public.[41] In either case, this kind of idea frequently meets itching ears on the part of the public and those who feel vindicated by the information and/or putative diagnoses, correct or not, they have received through DTC testing.

Overdiagnosis and the Cost of Follow-up

Incorrect diagnoses and inaccurate laboratory results are tenaciously sticky in the medical record. In the past, these were reviewed by medical students, residents, and staff physicians at each new medical encounter, which afforded an opportunity for selective revision. With the advent of the electronic health record, previous diagnoses are autopopulated into new encounter records and contribute to an ever-snowballing accretion of information accrued from the prior record. In short, it is difficult to purge an incorrect diagnosis from the medical record. Overdiagnosis, however, is not just a matter of error propagation. For example, patients with presumptive diagnosis of Lyme disease, whether they had experienced objective evidence of infection or not, use considerable medical resources in follow-up visits and are vulnerable to iatrogenic harm. In 1 study, patients were exposed to a median of 75 days of antibiotics if they had objective evidence of infection and 42 days of antibiotics, even in the absence of evidence of infection.[42] Medical and diagnostic interventions are not benign and have well-established complications. The complications of inappropriate antibiotic therapy for Lyme disease have included hepatic drug reactions, *Clostridium difficile*–associated diarrhea and colitis, thrombophlebitis, infections at the site of intravenous administration[42] and, in 1 rare case, death.[43]

In the case of genetic testing, the situation is similar. Although there is little dispute regarding the value of genetic testing for monogenic diseases in appropriate patient populations, this testing usually is performed as part of routine medical care. In a broader context of DTC genetic testing, however, some companies report increased or decreased risk of various medical conditions based on genome-wide association studies of single nucleotide genetic variants (so-called secondary findings). With these reports, which superficially appear to have many actionable findings, patients inevitably follow-up with their primary care giver for explanation and direction, not realizing that the primary care giver will, with rare exception, be equally unprepared to interpret and respond to the results. As McGuire and Burke[44] point out, if the testing suggests increased odds ratios for malignancy, which in some contexts may be as low as 1.5,[45] the physician may feel ethically or medical legally compelled to perform longitudinal surveillance with tumor marker testing, computed tomography, colonoscopy, and so forth. Furthermore, although many physicians and patients alike may consider genetic testing to be black and white because presence or absence of mutation is reported, the principles of false discovery still apply when pretest probabilities are low and the target variant is rare.[46,47]

Almost all physicians, including the author,[48] can relate stories of iatrogenic harm associated with subsequent interventions following-up abnormal diagnostic tests for which the initial indications were weak or absent. Not only are these abnormal findings a source of anxiety and potential harm to patients but also the DTC model raids the medical commons,[44] that is, it offloads all of the cost of downstream investigation and care onto the medical insurer, which in many countries is the public purse. Furthermore, although profiting on patients' health concerns, anxiety, or even curiosity, the risk of all pursuant invasive medical action falls onto patients and their medical caregivers, creating illness where there was none, furthering the risk of false discovery and consuming the physician human resource, which is chronically scarce.

UTILIZATION MANAGEMENT, CULTURE SHIFTS AND CONVERSATIONS

Financial pressure on the medical system and inappropriate or thoughtless use of diagnostic testing has led to targeted efforts to curtail low-utility testing through nationally funded efforts promoting rational test utilization, such as Choosing Wisely (CW).[49] Publications citing the CW initiative grew rapidly from 2014 to 2016 and now hold steady at approximately 120 per year (**Fig. 2**). Efforts to curtail inappropriate testing either algorithmically or by targeted rationing of certain conspicuously abused tests like 25-hydroxyvitamin D continue with some notable successes.[50] Paradoxically and contemporaneously, efforts in the field of personalized and precision medicine encourage pharmacogenomic/genetic/laboratory diagnostic entrepreneurism,[51] which in-turn drives testing for which there may be little to no indication. The fact

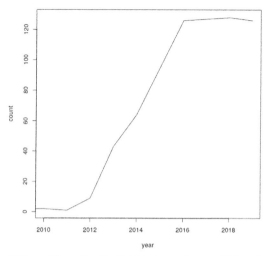

Fig. 2. Number of articles retrieved by the PubMed search term, "Choosing Wisely", by publication year.

that both CW and other resource-stewardship initiatives coexist in the same broader medical system as DTC testing is highly irrational and more or less corresponds to a medical system that is eating its own tail.

The smartwatch has created a culture where individuals collect information related to their health at all times, even in their sleep. These data inform them of their daily numbers of steps, flights of stairs, motions during sleep, and heart rate. Additionally, devices targeted to specific sports can provide stride length, speed, running/cycling cadence, power delivery, and elevation. Elaborate, automated computational analysis of these data can provide consumers with incentive for fitness improvement and allow them to chart their progress over time. It has been shown that these tools are effective at engaging adults in fitness improvement, although it amounts to gamification of training.[52]

For consumers exposed to the smartwatch, it seems natural that the same frequent or constant monitoring would be of benefit in other areas of their health—the attitude being, "If some data are good, more data are always better." Accordingly, entrepreneurs have sought to profit by offering tools for frequent monitoring of blood biomarkers of various medical conditions. Naturally, in some instances, the case for constant monitoring is entirely sensible—for example, in blood glucose sensors for diabetics. The reasoning as to why the same principles do not apply to all other diagnostic and genetic tests, however, is difficult for the general public to appreciate. Also at play is an apparent disregard for valuable low-tech and low-cost medical information: family history, weight, waist circumference, and blood pressure. Because the data revolution is not going away, it behooves primary care givers to explain to patients that some conditions benefit from constant monitoring and most distinctly do not.

Notwithstanding the competing pressures of an increasingly data-driven culture, the desire to support entrepreneurism for its economic benefits and the imminent need for cost containment through medical stewardship, the DTC market will continue to grow unless thwarted through regulation. This seems unlikely given the current state and the money to be made. For this reason, the primary care giver needs to be proactive in instructing patients who inquire about these services regarding the variable quality of the testing offered and the risk of experiencing more harm than good. Physicians should not respond dismissively, not only because it undermines patient trust but also because DTC testing companies tend to play on patients' frustrations with their primary care givers. Physicians also must be prepared to review unfamiliar genetic and multipanel biochemical diagnostic testing and maintain sufficient rapport that their critical evaluation can be heard. It is important for physicians to explain that the tests have uncertain and unproved diagnostic value. Showing patients statements from regulatory bodies also can provide helpful reinforcement. Ultimately, however, patients may be so invested in the notion they have discovered medical value in the DTC market that they cannot be dissuaded from their beliefs. In that context, clinicians are reminded that the best thing that can be done for patients is to tell them the truth, but it is not up to clinicians to make them believe it.

SUMMARY

Sir William Osler, the famous Canadian clinician and expert in laboratory medicine said, "As is our pathology so is our practice."[53] If diagnostic testing is freed from traditional constraints of the patient/doctor/pathologist relationship that keeps patients' welfare the primary aim while holding off the self-interested motives of outsiders, laboratory testing may become an entirely profit-driven Wild West. Consumers will be helpless to defend themselves against faulty products because they lack tools to evaluate the quality of the product. Downstream financial penalization of vendors will be delayed and only achievable at the cost of missed diagnoses and iatrogenic morbidity. The negative consequences of shoddy laboratory workmanship was exemplified by Theranos, which marketed itself as the emancipator of diagnostic medicine. But even if Theranos was able to provide high-quality DTC testing, as Osler also said, "A physician who treats himself has a fool for a patient."[54] In the DTC testing paradigm, it seems the free market is encouraging nonphysicians to treat themselves, making them doubly fooled.

DISCLOSURE

Dr D.T. Holmes provides clinical mass spectrometry consultation to Dian Diagnostics in Hangzhou, China.

REFERENCES

1. Clarke SF, Foster JR. A history of blood glucose meters and their role in self-monitoring of diabetes mellitus. Br J Biomed Sci 2012;69(2):83–93.
2. Vaitukatis JL. Development of the home pregnancy test. Ann N Y Acad Sci 2004; 1038(1):220–2.
3. Wallach EE, Corsan GH, Ghazi D, et al. Home urinary luteinizing hormone immunoassays: clinical applications. Fertil Steril 1990;53(4):591–601.
4. Gardiner C, Williams K, Mackie IJ, et al. Patient self-testing is a reliable and acceptable alternative to laboratory inr monitoring. Br J Haematol 2005;128(2): 242–7.
5. Ibitoye M, Frasca T, Giguere R, et al. Home testing past, present and future: lessons learned and implications for HIV home tests. AIDS Behav 2014;18(5): 933–49.
6. Grebely J, Applegate TL, Cunningham P, et al. Hepatitis c point-of-care diagnostics: in search of a single visit diagnosis. Expert Rev Mol Diagn 2017;17(12): 1109–15.

7. Patel MR, Hellkamp AS, Fox KAA. Point-of-care warfarin monitoring in the rocket af trial. N Engl J Med 2016;374(8):785–8.

8. Roche diagnostics recalls coaguchek Xs Pt test strips due to inaccurate Inr test results. White Oak, Maryland: US Food; Drug Administration; 2018. Available at: https://www.fda.gov/medical-devices/medical-device-recalls/roche-diagnostics-recalls-coaguchek-xs-pt-test-strips-due-inaccurate-inr-test-results. Accessed October 25, 2019.

9. Schulze M. 25 percent more states allow direct access testing. Lab Med 2001; 32(11):661–4.

10. Williams-Jones B. Where there'sa web, there's a way: commercial genetic testing and the internet. Community Genet 2003;6(1):46–57.

11. Allyse MA, Robinson DH, Ferber MJ, et al. Direct-to-consumer testing 2.0: emerging models of direct-to-consumer genetic testing. Mayo Clin Proc 2018; 93(1):113–20.

12. Topol E, Holmes E. Creative disruption? She's 29 and set to reboot lab medicine. Medscape; 2013. Available at: https://www.medscape.com/viewarticle/814233_6. Accessed October 25, 2019.

13. Parloff R. Theranos on the ropes as scathing regulatory report is made public. Fortune; 2016. Available at: https://fortune.com/2016/04/01/theranos-regulatory-report/. Accessed October 25, 2019.

14. Physician treatment of self, family members, or others close to them. Ontario, Canada: The College of Physicians; Surgeons of Ontario; 2018. Available at: https://www.cpso.on.ca/Physicians/Policies-Guidance/Policies/Physician-Treatment-of-Self-Family-Members-or. Accessed October 25, 2019.

15. Treating self or family: code of medical ethics opinion 1.2.1. Chicago, USA: The American Medical Association; 2019. Available at: https://www.ama-assn.org/delivering-care/ethics/treating-self-or-family. Accessed October 25, 2019.

16. Giardina TD, Modi V, Parrish DE, et al. The patient portal and abnormal test results: an exploratory study of patient experiences. Patient Exp J 2015;2(1):148.

17. Giardina TD, Baldwin J, Nystrom DT, et al. Patient perceptions of receiving test results via online portals: a mixed-methods study. J Am Med Inform Assoc 2017;25(4):440–6.

18. Deyo RA. Cascade effects of medical technology. Annu Rev Public Health 2002; 23(1):23–44.

19. Rigby AS. Statistical methods in epidemiology: I. Statistical errors in hypothesis testing. Disabil Rehabil 1998;20(4):121–6.

20. Morris Jane G, Swaraj S, Marc F. Testing for inherited thrombophilias in arterial stroke. Stroke 2019;41(12):2985–90.

21. Epner PL, Gans JE, Graber ML. When diagnostic testing leads to harm: a new outcomes-based approach for laboratory medicine. BMJ Qual Saf 2013; 22(Suppl 2):ii6. Available at: http://qualitysafety.bmj.com/content/22/Suppl_2/ii6.abstract.

22. DeKay ML, Asch DA. Is the defensive use of diagnostic tests good for patients, or bad? Med Decis Making 1998;18(1):19–28.

23. Deeks JJ, Altman DG. Diagnostic tests 4: likelihood ratios. Br Med J 2004; 329(7458):168–9.

24. Plebani M, Lippi G. Closing the brain-to-brain loop in laboratory testing. Clin Chem Lab Med 2019;49:1131. https://www.degruyter.com/view/j/cclm.2011.49.issue-7/cclm.2011.617/cclm.2011.617.xml.

25. Lundberg GD. Acting on significant laboratory results. JAMA 1981;245(17): 1762–3.

26. Marques AR. Lyme disease: a review. Curr Allergy Asthma Rep 2010;10(1): 13–20.
27. Steere AC, Batsford WP, Weinberg M, et al. Lyme carditis: cardiac abnormalities of lyme disease. Ann Intern Med 1980;93:8–16.
28. Pfister H-W, Rupprecht TA. Clinical aspects of neuroborreliosis and post-lyme disease syndrome in adult patients. Int J Med Microbiol 2006;296:11–6.
29. Group TIW. Evidence-based guidelines for the management of lyme disease. Expert Rev Anti Infect Ther 2004;2(sup1):S1–13.
30. Lantos PM. Chronic lyme disease: the controversies and the science. Expert Rev Anti Infect Ther 2011;9(7):787–97.
31. Buchwald D, Umali P, Umali J, et al. Chronic fatigue and the chronic fatigue syndrome: prevalence in a pacific northwest health care system. Ann Intern Med 1995;123(2):81–8.
32. Coulter I, Willis E. Explaining the growth of complementary and alternative medicine. Health Sociol Rev 2007;16(3–4):214–25.
33. Fallon BA, Pavlicova M, Coffino SW, et al. A comparison of lyme disease serologic test results from 4 laboratories in patients with persistent symptoms after antibiotic treatment. Clin Infect Dis 2014;59(12):1705–10.
34. Dattwyler RJ, Arnaboldi PM. Editorial commentary: comparison of lyme disease serologic assays and lyme specialty laboratories. Clin Infect Dis 2014;59(12): 1711–3.
35. Patrick DM, Complex Chronic Disease Study Group, Miller RR, et al. Lyme disease diagnosed by alternative methods: a phenotype similar to that of chronic fatigue syndrome. Clin Infect Dis 2015;61(7):1084–91.
36. Notice to readers recommendations for test performance and interpretation from the Second National Conference on Serologic Diagnosis of Lyme Diseases. Atlanta, USA: US Centers for Disease Control Prevention; 2019. Available at: https://www.cdc.gov/mmwr/preview/mmwrhtml/00038469.htm. Accessed October 25, 2019.
37. Paul Mead JP, Hinckley A. . Updated CDC recommendation for serologic diagnosis of Lyme diseases. US Centers for Disease Control; Prevention; 2019. Available at: https://www.cdc.gov/mmwr/volumes/68/wr/mm6832a4.htm?s_cid=mm 6832a4_ws.
38. B.J. Johnson, Laboratory diagnostic testing for *Borrelia burgdorferi* infection. In Lyme Disease: An Evidence-Based Approach 1st ed. edited by John J. Halperin. Centre for Agriculture and Bioscience International, Cambridge, USA. p. 73-88.
39. Webber B, Burganowski R, Colton L, et al. Lyme disease overdiagnosis in a large healthcare system: a population-based, retrospective study. Clin Microbiol Infect 2019. https://doi.org/10.1016/j.cmi.2019.02.020.
40. Lantos PM, Lipsett SC, Nigrovic LE. False positive lyme disease IgM immunoblots in children. J Pediatr 2016;174:267–9.e1.
41. Kosoff M. World's most loyal V.C. Says Theranos critics are just haters. Vanity Fair 2019. Available at: https://www.vanityfair.com/news/2016/06/worlds-most-loyal-vc-says-theranos-critics-are-just-haters. Accessed October 25, 2019.
42. Reid MC, Schoen RT, Evans J, et al. The consequences of overdiagnosis and overtreatment of lyme disease: an observational study. Ann Intern Med 1998; 128(5):354–62.
43. Patel R, Grogg KL, Edwards WD, et al. Death from inappropriate therapy for lyme disease. Clin Infect Dis 2000;31(4):1107–9.
44. McGuire AL, Burke W. An unwelcome side effect of direct-to-consumer personal genome testing: raiding the medical commons. JAMA 2008;300(22):2669–71.

45. Hunter DJ, Khoury MJ, Drazen JM. Letting the genome out of the bottle – will we get our wish? N Engl J Med 2019;358(2):105–7.
46. Predham S, Hamilton S, Elliott AM, et al. Case report: direct access genetic testing and a false-positive result for long qt syndrome. J Genet Couns 2015. https://doi.org/10.1007/s10897-015-9882-0.
47. Weedon MN, Jackson L, Harrison JW, et al. Very rare pathogenic genetic variants detected by snp-chips are usually false positives: implications for direct-to-consumer genetic testing. bioRxiv 2019;696–799.
48. Khan W, Van Der Gugten G, Holmes DT. Thyrotoxicosis due to 1000-fold error in compounded liothyronine: a case elucidated by mass spectrometry. Clin Mass Spectrom 2019;11:8–11.
49. Choosing wisely: promoting conversations between patients and clinicians. American Board of Internal Medicine; 2019. Available at: https://www.choosingwisely.org. Accessed October 25, 2019.
50. Naugler C, Hemmelgarn B, Quan H, et al. Implementation of an intervention to reduce population-based screening for vitamin d deficiency: a cross-sectional study. CMAJ Open 2017;5(1):E36.
51. Diamandis EP. Theranos phenomenon: promises and fallacies. Clin Chem Lab Med 2015;53(7):989–93.
52. Cadmus-Bertram LA, Marcus BH, Patterson RE, et al. Randomized trial of a fitbit-based physical activity intervention for women. Am J Prev Med 2015;49(3):414–8.
53. Osler W. An address on the treatment of disease: being the address in medicine before the ontario medical association, toronto, june 3rd, 1909. Br Med J 1909; 2(2534):185.
54. Osler W, Bennet R, Bennet W. Sir William Osler: Aphorisms from His Bedside Teachings and Writings. New York: Henry Schuman, Inc.; 1950. Available at: https://archive.org/details/in.ernet.dli.2015.63933/page.

Big Data Everywhere
The Impact of Data Disjunction in the Direct-to-Consumer Testing Model

Emily L. Gill, PhD[a], Stephen R. Master, MD, PhD[a,b],*

KEYWORDS

- Big Data • Laboratory medicine • Machine learning • Direct-to-consumer testing
- DTC • Harmonization

KEY POINTS

- Big Data and machine-learning approaches to analytics are an important new frontier in laboratory medicine.
- Direct-to-consumer (DTC) testing raises specific challenges in applying these new tools of data analytics.
- Because DTC data are not centralized by default, there is a need for data repositories to aggregate these values to develop appropriate predictive models.
- The lack of a default linkage between DTC results and medical outcomes data also limits the ability to mine these data for predictive modeling of disease risk.
- Issues of standardization and harmonization, which are a significant issue across all laboratory medicine, may be particularly difficult to correct in aggregated sets of DTC data.

BIG DATA IN LABORATORY MEDICINE

The past 20 years have produced an exponential increase in the amount of stored digital data, with some estimates claiming that the total amount worldwide will reach 40 trillion gigabytes by 2020.[1] This situation has in turn created the phenomenon of "Big Data," a term that reflects the new technical and interpretive challenges that arise from data sets that are many orders of magnitude larger than those previously seen. Although the term may seem self-explanatory, references to Big Data in both the scientific literature and lay press appear to fall into at least three main categories: a technical definition in which Big Data is viewed primarily with reference to the technological challenges of storing and searching data repositories that are too large to be housed

[a] Department of Pathology and Laboratory Medicine, Children's Hospital of Philadelphia, Philadelphia, PA, USA; [b] Department of Pathology and Laboratory Medicine, University of Pennsylvania, Perelman School of Medicine, Philadelphia, PA, USA
* Corresponding author. Children's Hospital of Philadelphia, 34th and Civic Center Boulevard, Room 5145, Philadelphia, PA 19104-4399.
E-mail address: masters@email.chop.edu

Clin Lab Med 40 (2020) 51–59
https://doi.org/10.1016/j.cll.2019.11.009
0272-2712/20/© 2019 Elsevier Inc. All rights reserved.

on a single computer or storage device; a functional definition, referring to particular characteristics of emerging data sets such as volume, velocity, variety, and veracity[2]; and an analytical definition, referring to the need to use high-dimensional data analysis and machine-learning tools to adequately interpret and use the data. Although many medical data sets may face the challenges imposed by the technical and functional definitions, the analytical definition seems to best encapsulate the shared approaches and promise of data analytics in laboratory medicine.

The advent of so-called Big Data has revolutionized a number of industries, with some of its most successful commercial applications arising in the realm of predictive analytics for consumer behavior. The increasing amount of information collected via Web browsing and social media activity, for example, can be used to target advertising in an increasingly effective way, despite the potential complexity of the incoming data. Similarly, as laboratory data have become more plentiful both at a single time point (with increased numbers of conventional tests or newer, highly multiplexed testing formats) and across time (with longitudinal testing), there is increased enthusiasm for using the same tools of machine learning that have been so successfully applied in the commercial sphere to provide more effective disease detection. As one example, integrated analysis of medical and laboratory data sets has recently been reported by multiple groups to significantly improve the early detection of acute kidney injury in a hospital setting.[3–5] Such encouraging results will, no doubt, accelerate efforts to further use machine learning with "big" laboratory data to improve patient care. Importantly, these encouraging results are possible because research groups have linked access to both the primary predictive variables (medical and laboratory data) and the clinical outcomes.

At the same time as laboratory data sets are increasing in size and value, direct-to-consumer (DTC) testing[6] has emerged as a possible additional stream of data that may contribute to health care diagnostics. The fundamentals of DTC testing are covered in detail elsewhere in this issue, but it is worth emphasizing that one argument for increased DTC access has come from the so-called quantitative self movement,[7] which argues that increased data collection and subsequent analysis may fundamentally improve the ability for an individual patient to understand and predict the state of their health. This type of analysis would, presumably, rely heavily on the type of Big Data analytics that we have described to interpret the raw test values over time, and—as such—shares common concerns with other applications of machine learning using traditional (non-DTC) sources of laboratory data.

Given this emerging shared interest in Big Data approaches, it is worth asking whether there are unique challenges posed to high-dimensional, machine-learning approaches when using DTC data. Specifically, what are the unique aspects of DTC data that are different from non-DTC laboratory data, and how will we need to account for these when developing novel interpretive tools for understanding patient health?

COLLECTING DIRECT-TO-CONSUMER TEST DATA

The first issue in assessing the feasibility of Big Data analytics using DTC test results is determining their availability and centralization. As the DTC field is currently fragmented and evolving more rapidly than the more stable, peer-reviewed literature, any assessment of its current state is only an approximation. Nonetheless, it is important to make some assessment of data availability.

Table 1 lists a variety of current DTC-testing providers and their mechanisms for returning results. The most common delivery method is electronic access via a password-protected portal, although a few providers provide other alternatives

Table 1
Ten established direct-to-consumer testing companies

Service Provider	Tests Offered	Procedure	Results	MD Referral
23andMe (https://www.23andme.com/)	Health predisposition Wellness reports Carrier status Other	Consumers order the test online and receive an at-home kit to send in a saliva sample for analysis	Results are sent to the patient's password-protected account	No
Any Lab Test Now (https://www.anylabtestnow.com/)	General health Sexual health Other	Consumers choose a test and make an on-site appointment	Results can be emailed (test dependent), mailed, faxed, or collected in person	No
Health Check USA (http://www.healthcheckusa.com/)	Cancer screening Hormone testing Sexual health Other	Consumers order their test online and visit a testing center	Results are made available online through a password-protected portal when available	No
Direct Laboratory Service (https://www.directlabs.com/)	Heart health Cancer screening Hormone testing Other	Consumers order their test online and attend an on-site appointment	Results are received through a password-protected online portal	No
My Med Lab (https://www.mymedlab.com/)	Allergy screening Cancer screening Blood disorders Other	Consumers order their test online and a "My Med Lab" MD approves the request. Consumers visit a testing site	Results are available online through a password-protected portal	No
Laboratory Corporation of America (https://www.pixel.labcorp.com/)	Kidney health Thyroid testing Metabolic panel Other	Consumers make an appointment for a specific test online and attend an on-site appointment	Results are available online through a password-protected portal	Yes[a]
Quest Diagnostics Inc. (https://www.questdiagnostics.com)	General health Heart health Sexual health Other	Consumers order a test online and attend an on-site appointment	Results are available online through a password-protected portal when available	Yes[a]
Sonora Quest Lab (https://www.sonoraquest.com/)	General health Allergy screening Digestive health Other	Consumers order the test online and attend an on-site appointment. At-home phlebotomy is also available	Results are available online through a password-protected portal, by email, fax, mail, or in-person collection	No

(continued on next page)

				MD
Service Provider	**Tests Offered**	**Procedure**	**Results**	**Referral**
Walk in Lab (https://www.walkinlab.com/)	Diabetes testing Sexual health Hormone testing Other	Consumers make an appointment for a specific test online and attend an on-site appointment	Results are available online through a password-protected portal	No
Pathway Genomics (https://www.pathway.com/)	Mental health Heart health Carrier status Other	Consumers order their test online and receive an at-home kit. A cheek swab is mailed back for analysis	Results are available online through a password-protected portal when available	Yes[a]

Table 1
(continued)

[a] Physician-ordering and DTC-testing company.

including mail, in-person reporting, and delivery directly to an MD provider. Generally, the consumers themselves must in some way (Web- or app-based) access the data and retrieve it in an interpretable form. This is consistent with one of the main arguments for DTC testing, namely, that it not only allows the patient to control which tests are ordered, but also to determine whether and with whom the information is shared. In the case of certain results (such as drugs of abuse or testing for sexually transmitted diseases) that may be considered to hold the potential for social stigma, one argument in favor of the DTC approach rather than an MD-mediated approach is that it gives the patient maximal control over his or her own sensitive information.[8]

It is worth contrasting this approach with other trends in the dissemination of medical data within the current United States health care system. Since the advent of increased privacy protection under the Health Insurance Portability and Accountability Act of 1996 (HIPAA) and the safeguards that it provides, there has been a reasonable presumption that increased dissemination of medical information within HIPAA-compliant settings provides a benefit for patient health. Not only is this the case within an individual medical system, where multiple providers have access to a patient's medical record to provide timely and optimal care, it is now even the case (with patient consent) between independent medical systems that use the same electronic medical record (EMR) provider and thus can seamlessly transmit the most up-to-date patient information as required for treatment.

This ability to aggregate large amounts of medical data is not only important for cross-system patient care but also raises the possibility of improving population health by understanding the relationship between laboratory results and patient outcomes in Big-Data-sized cohorts. With individual consent, Institutional Review Board waiver, or the use of deidentified data, it is possible to use such large data repositories to generate machine-learning models that better predict disease incidence or prognosis. By using such models, a patient or health care provider can potentially receive more helpful information to understand health status or guide treatment. Arguably, by analogy with the use of Big Data in commercial applications, it is precisely this improved use of analytics that has led to an expectation that increasing the variety or frequency of testing will result in improved patient health.

However, the current state of DTC testing leads to some obvious challenges for this model. First, with the exception of the minority of DTC laboratories that return results directly to clinicians, any integration of most DTC results into large data cohorts will require patients to take the initiative to centralize such results themselves. Exercising control over one's own data (and particularly medical data) is, of course, an important aspect of individual autonomy; indeed, it is a foundational principle of medical ethics. However, in the absence of a seamless way to transmit such results to a central data repository that adequately protects patient privacy (at least to the degree that HIPAA-regulated EMRs do so), the development of predictive models to help patients interpret the medical meaning of their data may be slower than it would be otherwise. Second, the potentially selective reporting of such data in a systematic way (such as when there is social stigma) carries with it the potential for confounding and ascertainment bias in any resulting model. It will be important for data scientists attempting to build medically valid predictive models from DTC results to be particularly cognizant of this issue.

OUTCOMES LINKAGE

A second challenge to the use of DTC results for Big Data analytics follows directly from this first issue of data centralization. A potential solution to the problem of fragmented data is, as already suggested, to provide a convenient, centralized portal for patients to enter their results so that they can be used to generate models that may, in the future, provide interpretive benefits for the patients themselves. This centralized portal could be provided by a governmental (e.g., National Institutes of Health), nonprofit, or commercial provider. If any one group was able to capture a significant fraction of the data with well-described protocols, there might be sufficient incentive for DTC providers to create a more streamlined way for consumers to directly upload their data to the centralized portal. By analogy, it seems that some commercial providers are already thinking in these terms, and have created ways for patients to transfer their existing EMR information into the commercial entity's database (e.g., the Apple Health App[9]). This allows centralization within this commercial database. Conversely, if the DTC data exist in a commercial database, transfer to a traditional EMR would integrate them into the conventional medical system. Indeed, even the inclusion of consumer medical results in the EMR has previously been described.[10] Approaches that seamlessly transfer DTC data to the traditional medical record have the potential added advantage of ensuring that patient results are accurately provided to a clinician.

Leaving aside considerations of how the commercial aspects of such a portal might be handled while ensuring equitable access, however, it is important to consider the requirements for any successful data repository when creating predictive analytics. Most significantly, Big Data analytical approaches to laboratory medicine require not only the laboratory results themselves but also appropriate clinical data and outcomes that should be linked with them. By analogy, the success of commercial enterprises such as Amazon and Netflix in using Big Data approaches to predict consumer behavior is based precisely on their ability to combine (imperfect) predictive data with significantly more complete outcomes data (e.g., which products were actually purchased from Amazon, or which movie was chosen on Netflix).

This is the primary reason why the DTC companies themselves are often not well poised to create predictive machine-learning models: lack of appropriate medical context and follow-up. For example, although 23andMe have acquired SNP (single-nucleotide polymorphism) genotyping data at a population scale, their ability to use those data to generate medical interpretation beyond that which exists in the medical literature depends on patients providing additional phenotypic information via voluntary questionnaires. Indeed, it is linkage of primary laboratory and medical data to outcomes within large medical centers and systems that has led to many of the most successful uses of Big Data within a diagnostic context (such as the acute kidney injury studies referenced earlier).

To address this challenge, it is important that any aggregation of DTC data be undertaken in a context that will also acquire sufficient outcomes data. Ideally, such outcomes should be ascertained and coded in a way that maximizes comparability. Although even individual health systems often do not achieve this goal, the level of diagnostic comparability achieved in such settings can provide a useful initial target. In fact, providing more streamlined ways for patients to transfer results into their current EMR (without requiring manual transcription by either the patient or provider) might be the most efficient initial step to integrate DTC results into an existing framework for collecting outcomes data.

STANDARDIZATION AND HARMONIZATION

A third challenge for using DTC results in Big Data approaches arises from an issue that affects a wide variety of assays in laboratory medicine: standardization and harmonization. Although the terminology is currently evolving, standardization traditionally referred to agreement between assays for which a reference material and methodology exist (whereby the assays can be assessed against a "gold standard"), and harmonization referred to achieving a consensus between assays for which no such "gold standard" exists.[11] In either case, the fundamental issue is that assays obtained from different manufacturers or that represent different methodologies may not necessarily yield the same results.

It has long been recognized that this problem can have a significant impact on patient care, particularly when there are national guidelines that recommend changes in treatment based on cutoff values.[12] A significant amount of international work has focused on correcting these issues, with a particular focus on single analytes that are known to carry such an impact on patient care. When considering multivariate machine-learning models derived from Big Data, however, it is less clear whether such efforts have been sufficient. Rather than focusing on known, medically significant analytes, these high-dimensional models may capture previously unknown interactions between variables that determine, for instance, medical risk; as such, it is more difficult to determine a priori which are likely to require significant harmonization.

The effects of bias between test platforms can be mitigated when the Big Data results are obtained from a single medical center or central laboratory using a uniform testing methodology. Although such models may or may not necessarily be directly portable to other measurement platforms, within an individual laboratory it can be relatively more straightforward to detect complex relationships and build a reliable model. By contrast, building predictive machine-learning models using laboratory data obtained with nonharmonized assays across multiple sites is fundamentally more challenging, particularly if there is a confounding relationship between measurement bias at a given site and disease prevalence.

To comprehensively address the challenges of incomplete standardization and harmonization, investigators must know both the specific assay used to generate each individual result and the relationship between that assay and others that measure the same analyte within patient specimens. This challenge exists regardless of whether the results are delivered in a DTC context. In the case of data derived from combinations of large cohorts tested at a comparatively small number of laboratories, determining the association between an individual patient and the platform on which their testing was performed may be a manageable problem; however, when aggregating DTC results from patients who may have used a variety of DTC-testing sources over a period of time (and potentially different DTC laboratories for different analytes), the logistical challenges are significant.

One possible solution to this problem can be found by recognizing that, for common tests, most results are obtained from a relatively more constrained number of assays approved by the Food and Drug Administration. In such cases, it might be possible to combine results for patients based on their use of the same testing platform, regardless of the particular laboratory that performed the test. This approach would require two new developments. First, laboratories would need to routinely report the test platform used along with the results. Specific information on the manufacturer, model, and other factors will likely be required, as general parameters that can be modified based on local factors (such as reference range) will be insufficient to adequately correct the results. Second, any central repository that accepts these data will ideally need to store the same information in a form that will be amenable to future data mining and model building. These two considerations, however, could markedly improve the usability of DTC data for machine learning.

One significant objection to the aforementioned considerations, however, is that they fail to account for the prior success of Big Data approaches in the face of known problems with data veracity (sometimes called the fourth "V" of what we have referred to as the functional definition). By virtue of volume and velocity, Big Data analytics may be less sensitive to data-quality issues than when the same analytical approaches are performed on smaller data sets. There is certainly merit to this objection, and indeed there are significant examples of successful medical analytics derived from non-DTC, Big Data sources where there has been no explicit correction for standardization and harmonization. Indeed, one might argue that a major advantage of Big Data is that subpopulation biases become less important with a sufficiently large data sample, yielding a classifier that is appropriate under a wide variety of circumstances.

There are two important points when responding to this objection, however. First, although the lack of perfect data should not keep investigators from producing useful models, it is nevertheless true that creating the most accurate achievable predictive models is the goal for patient care. With traditional laboratory results obtained from one or a constrained number of testing centers or platforms, the location of those laboratory records remains an important link that can, in principle, be used to determine whether there is bias in the model based on the testing site. With DTC results, however, where the patients themselves represent the integrating point that passes the data along to a repository, such information is likely to be lost if it is not specifically collected and retained. Second, although clinicians working with laboratory values typically interpret them within a broader clinical context, a consumer who is directly using a machine-learning model using personal DTC data may not appreciate the potential effect of nonharmonized assays on the predictive results. The lack of clinical integration for DTC data managed solely by patients can raise the stakes of this problem compared with a traditional, physician-mediated interpretive model.

SUMMARY: THE FUTURE OF BIG DATA ANALYSIS FOR DIRECT-TO-CONSUMER TESTING

The advent of DTC testing provides significantly increased freedom for patients to control their medical testing and the dissemination of its results. Although there are important caveats to the use of DTC testing that are discussed elsewhere in this issue, most health care providers would likely agree that when and if these results can be translated into actionable, timely diagnostic information to improve health, this will be a positive development.

At the same time, the rapid increase in the amount of readily available medical and laboratory data has raised the possibility of significantly improving the laboratory community's ability to provide integrative, interpretive diagnosis through machine-learning algorithms to predict disease incidence and prognosis. The success of machine-learning techniques in the Big Data realms of commercial prediction of consumer behavior has increased the optimism that these same approaches will revolutionize health care. As indicated earlier, predictive analytics have already begun to show promising results in this arena.

However, as already discussed, specific aspects of the DTC paradigm present challenges to its successful incorporation into predictive models.

- Lack of centralized data repositories will hamper the development of any generalizable models, and the authors argue that this issue should be addressed in a manner that minimizes the barrier to patients in making their results available for developing such models (which, in turn, can increase the future predictive value of their data).
- Linking the data to outcomes is crucial for future analytical development, and migrating DTC data into the existing EMR may provide one seamless way to accomplish this.
- Standardization and harmonization can have a particular impact on data sets that aggregate DTC testing, when there is often a less direct link between testing methodology and results than is traditionally the case in data sets derived from one or a few large medical centers. Ongoing effort in the field is required.

The authors argue that addressing each of these challenges is important for maximizing the future value of DTC data.

Clinical laboratory medicine is a constantly evolving field, and new paradigms for ordering, generating, and reporting results will inevitably alter the way in which health care is delivered. As machine-learning analysis of Big Data represents one of the most exciting modern developments in our ability to improve the value of medical information, it is vital that as clinicians we consider the effect of new testing paradigms. By understanding the potential pitfalls and designing systems that allow us to overcome them, we will maximize our ability to navigate current trends in a way that maximizes the benefit to patients.

DISCLOSURE

The authors have nothing to disclose.

REFERENCES

1. Gantz J, Reinsel D. The digital universe in 2020: big data, bigger digital shadows, and biggest growth in the far east. 2012. IDC iView: IDC Analyze the Future. https://www.emc.com/leadership/digital-universe/2012iview/index.htm.

2. Gandomi A, Haider M. Beyond the hype: big data concepts, methods, and analytics. Int J Inf Manage 2015;35:137–44.

3. Selby NM, Crowley L, Fluck RJ, et al. Use of electronic results reporting to diagnose and monitor AKI in hospitalized patients. Clin J Am Soc Nephrol 2012;7:533–40.

4. Tomašev N, Glorot X, Rae JW, et al. A clinically applicable approach to continuous prediction of future acute kidney injury. Nature 2019;572:116–9.

5. Chiofolo C, Chbat N, Ghosh E, et al. Automated continuous acute kidney injury prediction and surveillance: a random forest model. Mayo Clin Proc 2019;94: 783–92.

6. Li M, Diamandis EP, Grenache D, et al. Direct-to-consumer testing. Clin Chem 2017;63:635–41.

7. Ajana B. Digital health and the biopolitics of the quantified self. Digit Health 2017; 3:1–18.

8. Johnson CC, Kennedy C, Fonner V, et al. Examining the effects of HIV self-testing compared to standard HIV testing services: a systematic review and meta-analysis. J Int AIDS Soc 2017;20:21594.

9. North F, Chaudhry R. Apple HealthKit and health app: patient uptake and barriers in primary care. Telemed J E Health 2016;22:608–13.

10. Kumar RB, Goren ND, Stark DE, et al. Automated integration of continuous glucose monitor data in the electronic health record using consumer technology. J Am Med Inform Assoc 2016;23:532–7.

11. Greg Miller W, Myers GL, Lou Gantzer M, et al. Roadmap for harmonization of clinical laboratory measurement procedures. Clin Chem 2011;57:1108–17.

12. Vesper HW, Myers GL, Miller WG. Current practices and challenges in the standardization and harmonization of clinical laboratory tests. Am J Clin Nutr 2016; 104:907S–12S.

The Impact of Direct-to-Consumer Genetic Testing on Patient and Provider

Mary Beth Palko Dinulos, MD*, Stephanie E. Vallee, MS

KEYWORDS

- Direct-to-consumer genetic testing • 23andMe • GWAS • SNPs

KEY POINTS

- When direct-to-consumer (DTC) genetic testing results are delivered directly to the consumer, without the involvement of a physician or genetic counselor (GC), we often encounter misinterpretation and needless medical interventions or false reassurance.
- Receiving DTC test results without appropriate genetic counseling can be overwhelming and anxiety-producing for the consumer.
- Increasingly, we are seeing patients who have done DTC genetic testing in our genetics clinics for test interpretation, management guidance, and confirmatory genetic testing because neither the consumer nor the primary care physicians have specialized training to interpret the findings.
- Educating the consumer regarding DTC genetic testing in general, as well as their specific results, is time-consuming and taxing of genetics clinic resources. Often the time spent by the GC is not reimbursable.

INTRODUCTION

Direct-to-consumer (DTC) genetic testing debuted in the early 2000s and gave consumers access to their genetic information without the involvement of a physician or genetic counselor (GC).[1] Over the past 2 decades, there has been controversy surrounding the clinical validity, clinical utility, and regulation of DTC genetic testing.[2,3] In addition, results are delivered directly to the consumer (often over the Internet), without the involvement of a physician or GC. This often leads to misinterpretation of test results and needless medical interventions or false reassurance.[4] Increasingly, we are seeing these patients in our genetics clinics for test interpretation, management guidance, and confirmatory genetic testing.

Departments of Pediatrics and Pathology, Dartmouth-Hitchcock Medical Center, Lebanon, NH 03576, USA
* Corresponding author.
E-mail address: mbd@hitchcock.org

Clin Lab Med 40 (2020) 61–67
https://doi.org/10.1016/j.cll.2019.11.003
0272-2712/20/© 2019 Elsevier Inc. All rights reserved.

DTC genetic testing uses the power of genome-wide association studies (GWAS) to detect single nucleotide polymorphisms (SNPs) that appear to be associated with specific disease states in the general population. These SNPs are not mutations within genes that are known to convey disease. SNPs are single changes (variants) within the genome that may be associated with disease in the general population. An association between a particular genome variant and a disease does not necessarily mean that the presence of that variant in a given individual is clinically meaningful. Herein lies the issue with predicting a disease state in an individual using only SNPs.

Recently, 23andMe was given permission by the Food and Drug Administration to test for actual mutations within the genes for several genetic conditions, including breast cancer. However, they are only testing for very specific mutations within those genes and are not preforming full sequencing of the genes. Therefore, a "negative" test only means that it is negative for the several mutations tested. This result may lead to false reassurance for those who test "negative." In addition, because of the high false positive rate in this testing, the "positive" result may actually be incorrect and cause undue anxiety and potential harm to the patient.

DISCUSSION

DTC genetic testing has become mainstream testing in the past decade, with companies such as 23andMe offering carrier testing and ancestry determination. Proponents of DTC genetic testing note that there are potential advantages of this type of testing.[5] Certainly from the standpoint of a clinical geneticist, one benefit is the greater awareness of genetics in the general population and the increased accessibility to genetic testing. DTC genetic testing enables the consumer to become proactive in making his or her own health care decisions. It can be empowering to the consumer because it provides a means of gaining medical information without using the traditional medical system. Consumers have a greater sense of autonomy with this type of genetic testing. An additional benefit is the ability to preserve anonymity with DTC genetic testing. Ordering tests and receiving results directly over the Internet bypasses the medical record and allows for increased privacy of the information obtained.

However, several major issues have surfaced with DTC genetic testing.[2,3] First, the clinical validity of each individual test must be established before entry into the market. Ideally, the clinical *utility* of each test also should be established: the test must provide information that is helpful to the individual being tested (eg, diagnosis, treatment). Second, the quality of the tests and the laboratories performing these tests must be rigorously controlled. Most importantly, in my opinion, it is imperative to involve a health care professional in the testing process to provide pretest and posttest counseling, interpretation of test results, and guidance in posttest decision making.

Recently I was lecturing to the medical students on the topic of genetic testing in the clinical practice of medicine. One of the students asked how DTC genetic testing impacted my genetics practice. Did we have many patients who came to us with their test results asking for interpretation or management guidelines? Were we inundated with requests to review a patient's DTC test results? My answer was a resounding yes, and I shared the following example with them.

A 45-year-old woman was referred to the genetics clinic by her primary care physician for evaluation of a possible connective tissue disorder. Concern for a diagnosis of Ehlers-Danlos syndrome (EDS) was raised during adolescence because of her joint hypermobility and pain symptoms. She stated that she was seen for evaluation in her late teens and a diagnosis of classic EDS (cEDS) was made. Review of those records was not possible during her clinic visit. Several years ago, she was evaluated by an endocrinologist who also agreed that she had clinical symptoms concerning for EDS.

In the evaluation of individuals with possible heritable connective tissue disorders, we review that there are multiple types of EDS, as well as other well-described disorders, such as Marfan syndrome, Loeys-Dietz syndrome, and Stickler syndrome. Each condition has unique/specific features and varied medical management. During our evaluation of the patient, each condition was considered because management of each connective tissue disorder is different.

Based on her medical history, family history, and physical examination findings, she fulfilled the clinical diagnostic criteria for EDS, hypermobile type (hEDS). We explained that the diagnosis of hEDS remains clinical, as there currently exists no diagnostic genetic testing for this type of EDS. In addition, she had no signs or symptoms to suggest another connective tissue disorder. Because she had been previously told that she had cEDS, we reviewed the diagnostic criteria for cEDS and explained that she did not have the significant skin hyperextensibility or atrophic scarring that were required to make that clinical diagnosis. Therefore, in the absence of those skin findings, the diagnosis of cEDS was not deemed correct.

During her clinic visit, we spent time reviewing her diagnosis of hEDS and our recommended medical management, as published by the 2017 International Consortium.[6] We advised using the hEDS management guidelines and symptom-specific publications regarding management. We also reviewed the current *GeneReviews* article pertaining to hEDS and referred her to several online resources providing additional information and support regarding joint hypermobility disorders.

We reviewed the following recommendations with this patient:

1. Management of symptoms of hEDS following guidelines as described in the hEDS *GeneReviews* article.[7]
2. We advised aquatherapy as the preferred modality for physical therapy in patients with EDS.
3. We recommended pain care providers for her chronic pain, which is seen in the vast majority of individuals with hEDS, but rarely noted in other types of EDS.
4. *We did not recommend genetic testing for connective tissue disorders, as there is no genetic testing available for hEDS.*

The patient left the genetics clinic with information regarding her new diagnosis of hEDS. We told her to contact us if she ever had additional questions or concerns.

One year later, we received an e-mail from this patient, explaining that she had performed the 23andMe genetic testing and then ran the raw genetic data through Live-Wello. She had received a report listing she had several variants associated with different types of EDS: heterozygous COL1A1, multiple homozygous COL5A1, heterozygous COL5A2, and one homozygous gene COL3A1 with additional homozygous genes flagged for mitochondrial issues. Given this information she was requesting to come back into our clinic and receive genetic testing because she was concerned about her children and the decline in her health.

When we respond to patients regarding their DTC genetic testing results, we find we have to address many issues. We must explain DTC genetic testing in language that the patient can understand. It is important to state that results received from the DTC companies may not be correct, and always need to be confirmed in a clinical diagnostic testing laboratory. The GC wrote to the patient:

We can certainly appreciate the concern you have after receiving a report showing this many "variants" in genes that could appear to be relevant given your symptoms and diagnosis. First, we need to caution you that there are studies that show that these types of direct-to-consumer (DTC) genetic testing kits report out gene variants that, when tested at clinical diagnostic labs, are not real. When tested under strict control, the gene changes are not actually there. There was a recent publication in the medical literature that reviewed results from DTC testing and found a false positive rate of approximately 40%. That publication was referencing the portion of testing that is supposedly diagnostic genetic testing, such as cystic fibrosis carrier status or breast cancer mutations.

SNPs are normal variations in the genetic code. Most SNPs have no effect on development or health. SNPs may be associated with complex diseases in the general population, but are not typically meaningful for an individual. DTC genetic testing companies such as 23andMe, as well as third-party interpretation companies such as LiveWello, are using SNPs in the context of "disease causing," which is incorrect. The GC wrote to the patient:

We were not familiar with LiveWello when I received your note, so we went to their website to see what type of service they are offering. Quick review suggests that they would be providing you with a list of single nucleotide polymorphisms or "SNPs" from the genetic data from your 23andMe testing. Aside from the fact that the variants may not even be real, please note that SNPs can be NORMAL variations in the genetic code. While their website links you out to 12 resources about the genes in which the SNPs are located, they are not saying that these SNPs cause these conditions. So, I worry that their presentation of this data is misleading and causing undue concern.

When performing DTC genetic testing through a company such as 23andMe, genetic counseling is not included in the cost of the test. However, genetic counseling may be offered for an additional fee. Third-party interpretation of raw data from DTC companies such as 23andMe is available through Web sites such as LiveWello, which generate a gene variance report based on hundreds of thousands of SNPs. No genetic counseling is included in the data interpretation, and consumers can easily become overwhelmed and anxious regarding the results. The GC wrote to the patient:

Reading genes is like reading a chapter in a book. When we perform diagnostic clinical genetic sequencing, we are looking for typos in that chapter. This would be the change of a single letter that is different from the "normal" code. However, not all changes are pathogenic (disease causing) and, in fact, the vast majority are benign (normal). Let's say that along the COL3A1 gene for vascular EDS there is a position where the usual letter at that spot is A and LiveWello found that you have a T instead. Then consider that they may say that 55% of the population has the A but you are in the 45% of the population that has a T. That still does not matter. The T may be the lesser common of the two options at that location, but 45% of the population doesn't have vascular EDS due to this COL3A1 SNP. Even if we shift those numbers and it is 95% that have the A and 5% have T, it still would not be significant. The T is a SNP and would have a minor allele frequency (MAF) of either 45% or 5% in the examples I have given. LiveWello provides you with SNPs. A clinical diagnostic lab would never report that information because it is not diagnostically relevant.

So then, why do we care about SNPs? There are researchers that study SNPs to see if the presence of a pattern of SNPs could correlate with specific medical conditions. For example, there are publications where they use "genome-wide association studies" (GWAS) where they may find that a certain constellation of 5 or 10 or 20 SNPs has a higher association with a certain condition. These are "associations" and are not causative or diagnostic. It is one way that researchers are trying to learn more about the genetic contribution to conditions that are considered to be multifactorial, meaning that they are due to the combination of multiple genetic and environmental factors, rather than genetic conditions that are due to a pathogenic variant in a single gene. While we have not found a single gene that causes hEDS, we do expect that there is a single gene, based on inheritance patterns in families. It could certainly prove to be more complex than that, so we cannot be sure, but there is no evidence to suggest that we should use SNPs in this way.

My first suggestion for you is that you review the results of your LiveWello report and look at the MAFs for each of the SNPs that are listed. I would hope that they are providing you with that information, but if not, they appear to reference the dbSNP site, which should show that information. If the MAFs are even in the single digits, and certainly if they are above 5%, they are normal. If you find that there are any that have a frequency below 1%, first remember that it might not be real, but you could let me know the details and I could take a look at it for you. It may be that 23andMe or LiveWello offer genetic counseling services and we would also suggest that you take advantage of those services.

Patient access and resources are very limited in medical genetics. Wait times for appointments may exceed 6 to 12 months at many academic centers. The number of individuals seeking genetic counseling for DTC genetic testing result interpretation far outweighs the availability of GCs. Insurance companies may not approve confirmatory genetic testing for these DTC results, depending on the circumstances surrounding the testing. The genetic counselor wrote to the patient:

We won't plan on making an appointment because our clinic honestly could not possibly follow-up on this type of testing for patients and there continues to be no clinical diagnostic testing available for hEDS. Even though we know there can be overlap between some of these connective tissue disorders, when we have any concern for rare forms of EDS (particularly anything that suggests vascular EDS) and sometimes in other rare situations where family history raises red flags (e.g., personal history of fractures or family history of aneurysms), we recommend genetic testing. In your clinic note, after examination and review of your history and symptoms, we stated that there is no genetic testing indicated. There are labs that offer EDS gene panels that include varying numbers of genes and at highly variable pricing. However, diagnostic genetic testing was not recommended, so we would not be able to obtain insurance coverage for this testing and your 23andMe/LiveWello results do not suggest that diagnostic testing is needed. Even when we have medical justification to do so, frankly, this testing may not be covered by many insurance companies.

Receiving "genetic testing results" from DTC companies without proper genetic counseling regarding the significance of the results can cause undue stress on the patient. In extreme cases the results may have untoward effects on patient management. For example, if an individual receives a "positive" breast/ovarian cancer gene result from a DTC company, they may opt for radical medical or surgical management, when in fact the result is a false positive. Alternatively, if the patient receives a "negative" result, but really has an increased risk of breast cancer, they may choose to forego proper surveillance.

However, back to our understanding of your personal concern for yourself and your children… We feel that you should know that there is a lab that offers clinical diagnostic genetic testing for EDS that involves comprehensive analysis of 15 genes that are known to cause some of the subtypes of EDS (including the ones you have mentioned, such as COL1A1, COL1A2, COL3A1, COL5A1, and COL5A2) and, when patients want to direct pay, they limit patient out-of-pocket costs to $250 (some EDS panels are 5–10 times that amount). It is an excellent lab, we use them regularly, and their goal is to make reliable, diagnostic genetic testing available. If they were to find a pathogenic gene variant, their policy is also to include follow-up diagnostic testing at no charge in ANY/ALL first degree relatives (parents, siblings, children) as long as family member samples are received within a couple of months of initial reporting. As I explained previously, we do not recommend genetic testing, as your history and examination findings are entirely consistent with hEDS, having fulfilled the requisite clinical diagnostic criteria. We would not expect to find clinically significant results and acknowledge that we could even further raise anxiety if the lab found a gene variant that is classified as being of uncertain clinical significance. The lab to which I refer is not DTC testing, so it requires a physician order to arrange this testing. In recognizing your anxiety and concern over this, if you choose, we can place an order for the panel through their direct ordering portal. They would ship you a saliva (spit) collection kit to send the sample back to them for testing but you would need to provide direct payment information with your sample.

I'm not sure if my explanation of 23andMe and LiveWello results will offer you sufficient reassurance or not, but I hope that it does.

Please let me know what you think.

SUMMARY

There are several important teaching points regarding our interaction with this patient following her DTC genetic testing. First, the time spent by the GC in response to this patient's inquiry was threefold greater than her initial clinic visit. This time was not billable. Had the patient actually come for an additional office visit, we could have billed for our services, but patient access and resources are very limited in medical genetics and we must prioritize access based on patient acuity.

When the patient left her initial clinic visit, she was reassured that she had hEDS, which does not have increased mortality. After receiving her DTC testing results, she had significant anxiety based on the ambiguity of the results, and her misunderstanding that she had a more serious form of EDS. She had no genetic counseling regarding these results and was fearful that her health and the health of her children may be compromised.

Clearly, the consumer's lack of health literacy complicates this whole process and may lead to increased anxiety and needless medical interventions based on erroneous or misinterpreted test results that indicate increased or decreased risk of disease. The DTC testing companies are reporting SNPs, which may show association with disease, but are not diagnostically relevant for an individual patient. This fact was never explained to the patient, as genetic counseling was not included in the cost of the testing.

Last, the false positive rate for some DTC genetic testing companies has been reported as high as 40%.[8] Therefore, results received from the DTC companies may not be correct, and always need to be confirmed in a clinical diagnostic testing laboratory, especially if the results will be used for clinical decision making.

For all of these reasons, in my opinion, DTC testing is not appropriate for diagnostic genetic testing at this time, and may even be detrimental to consumers. As per the American College of Medical Genetics and Genomics policy statement on DTC genetic testing, "… genetic testing should be provided to the public only through the services of an appropriately qualified health professional, who should be responsible for both ordering and interpreting the test, as well as for pretest and posttest counseling of individuals and families regarding the medical significance of test results and the need, if any, for follow-up."[3]

REFERENCES

1. Allyse MA, Robinson DH, Ferber MJ, et al. Direct-to-consumer testing 2.0: emerging models of direct-to-consumer genetic testing. Mayo Clin Proc 2018; 93(1):113–20.
2. Hudson K, Javitt G, Burke W, et al. ASHG statement on direct-to-consumer genetic testing in the United States. Obstet Gynecol 2007;110:1392–5.
3. ACMG. ACMG statement on direct-to-consumer genetic testing. Genet Med 2004; 6:60.
4. McGuire AL, Burke W. An unwelcome side effect of direct-to-consumer personal genome testing: raiding the medical commons. JAMA 2008;300(22):2669–71.
5. McBride CM, Wade C, Kaphingst KA. Consumers' view of direct-to-consumer genetic information. Annu Rev Genomics Hum Genet 2010;11:427–46.
6. Malfait F, Francomano C, Byers P, et al. The 2017 international classification of the Ehlers-Danlos syndromes. Am J Med Genet C Semin Med Genet 2017; 175(1):8–26.
7. Levy HP. Hypermobile Ehlers-Danlos syndrome. In: Adam MP, Ardinger HH, Pagon RA, et al, editors. GeneReviews®. Seattle (WA): University of Washington, Seattle; 2018. p. 1993–2019. Available at: https://www.ncbi.nlm.nih.gov/books/NBK1279/.
8. Tandy-Connor S, Guiltinan J, Krempely K, et al. False-positive results released by direct-to-consumer genetic tests highlight the importance of clinical confirmation testing for appropriate patient care. Genet Med 2018;20(12):1515–21.

Wave of Wearables

Clinical Management of Patients and the Future of Connected Medicine

Jeffrey Tully, MD[a],*, Christian Dameff, MD[b,c,d],
Christopher A. Longhurst, MD[e,f]

KEYWORDS

- Wearable electronic devices • Biosensors • Diagnostics • Drug delivery
- Personalized medicine • Telemedicine • Health monitoring

KEY POINTS

- Technologic advancement in health care continues to drive the expansion of health data. These data are increasingly being collected by devices called wearables.
- Existing literature focusing on wearables describe applications of novel technologies but lack outcomes data. Additional large-scale clinical trials are needed to show whether wearables are able to improve health outcomes or decrease health care costs.
- Efforts to reduce health care costs, increase care quality, and improve clinician efficiency are driving the development and study of wearables in medicine.
- The widespread use of wearables in clinical practice will depend on data integration with the electronic health record and physician workflow.

INTRODUCTION

Modern health care depends on technology across the care continuum. Value-based care incentives are facilitating a further expansion into consumer health. This process has been accompanied by a rapid expansion of health data, and the corresponding development of clinical informatics as a discipline dedicated to organizing, understanding, and using data to improve health care and patient outcomes.[1,2]

[a] Department of Anesthesiology and Pain Medicine, University of California Davis Medical Center, 2315 Stockton Boulevard, Sacramento, CA 95817, USA; [b] Department of Emergency Medicine, University of California San Diego, 200 West Arbor Drive #8676, San Diego, CA 92103, USA; [c] Department of Biomedical Informatics, UC San Diego Health, University of California San Diego, 9500 Gilman Drive, MC 0728, La Jolla, California 92093-0728, USA; [d] Department of Computer Science and Engineering, University of California San Diego, 9500 Gilman Drive, Mail Code 0404, La Jolla, CA 92093-0404, USA; [e] Department of Medicine, University of California San Diego, 9500 Gilman Drive, La Jolla, CA 92093, USA; [f] Department of Pediatrics, University of California San Diego, 9500 Gilman Drive, La Jolla, CA 92093, USA
* Corresponding author.
E-mail address: jltully@ucdavis.edu

Clin Lab Med 40 (2020) 69–82
https://doi.org/10.1016/j.cll.2019.11.004
0272-2712/20/© 2019 Elsevier Inc. All rights reserved.

The ubiquity of digital health increases opportunities to capture patient information derived outside the walls of a medical facility. The personal health record (PHR) is one way of integrating health data for individual patients across a multitude of environments.[3]

An increasingly prevalent source of data is the information generated by the subset of consumer technology known as wearable devices.[4] Broadly defined, wearable devices are specialized devices comprising a specialized sensor (or sensors) with a computer at a scale small enough to be worn or carried by individuals. This functionality may include the ability to measure or sense a certain physical parameter, or to provide a certain input or information to the user.[5] Many wearable devices feature the ability to connect wirelessly to other devices, facilitating the transfer and exchange of information and placing these devices in a category of technology known as the Internet of Things (IoT).[6]

This article provides a review of the clinical application, utility, or potential offered by a variety of commercially available wearable devices and technologies across several medical specialties in order to show the current and coming impact of these tools on the practice of medicine. This article excludes devices from the related, but more restricted, collection of medical devices ordered and prescribed under the direction of a clinician, such as a cardiac pacemaker. The latter category, designed for explicit therapeutic purposes, is required to engage in regulatory processes with the US Food and Drug Administration (FDA) in order to arrive to market,[7] whereas regulation for consumer devices offering a broad suite of functionality, both health and non–health related, is not as mature.[8] Although most wearable devices are currently marketed with the intention of being used by the consumer for largely self-directed activities, this article also discusses the use of these technologies in the setting of clinician-patient co-management and use.

USABILITY OF WEARABLE DEVICES

Literature focusing on the clinical impact and management of patients with wearable devices is limited. Peer-reviewed reports of novel applications of individual technologies outnumber clinical trials showing improved patient outcomes. Many investigators predict that the widespread adoption of this technology could lower health care costs through disease prevention and longitudinal care, although cost savings attributed to focused implementation of wearables have not been widely described.[9–12] Levine[13] proposes with several case studies that the technical simplicity, low production costs, and near ubiquity of wearable devices offer a particular potential for improving health in high-poverty and vulnerable populations.

Cross-sectional survey studies of primary care providers suggest they perceive benefits and trust wearable sensors and devices.[14,15] Patients also express openness to incorporating wearable sensors as part of health monitoring protocols, according to similarly constructed survey studies. However, consumers report opposition to wearable devices that are disruptive to daily life, or seen to replace traditional care provided by clinical professionals.[16] Several studies examine the aging geriatric population as a particular group that may benefit from an increased use of wearable technologies for medication management, prevention of falls, and monitoring of chronic disease,[17] although a relative decrease in ability to adopt new technology relative to younger generations has been cited as a potential barrier.[18]

Electronic health record (EHR) integration of wearable data is clearly advantageous to provider workflow.[19,20] Ryu and colleagues[21] developed a mobile application that received data from a variety of wearable sensors measuring activity and sleep data, and forwarded information into electronic medical record (EMR) platforms that clinicians then used to provide lifestyle and health counseling recommendations to target outcomes related to nutrition and obesity. Weenk and colleagues[22] presented a pilot study featuring wireless remote monitoring wearable devices collecting vital signs for patients in the inpatient setting, with the hypothesis that the continuous monitoring functionality represented an improvement compared with intermittent provider checks, which may contribute to earlier detection of deleterious changes in vital signs. The study focused on the ViSi Mobile (Sotera Wireless, San Diego, CA) and Health-Patch (Vital Connect, San Jose, CA) systems, capable of measuring and recording electrocardiogram (ECG), heart rate, respiratory rate, temperature, blood pressure, and oxygen saturation, and ECG, heart rate, respiratory rate, temperature, fall detection, and activity metrics, respectively. Indicators of patient and nurse acceptance of these monitoring systems were largely favorable. Lack of correlation between data reported by the devices and traditional bedside patient measurements by nurses was reported and attributed to measurement artifact and unreliable connectivity. Joshi and colleagues[23] reviewed a variety of similar patient vital monitoring platforms and provided additional commentary on considerations for the design of future trials.

The emergence of interoperable PHR platforms developed by the same producers of devices with health functionality suggests a trend toward comprehensive ecosystems in which consumer patients have increased accessibility to their personal health information, which preliminary data suggest may improve patient engagement with their health care providers.[24] Work using machine learning to analyze longitudinal data uploaded to EMRs from health care IoT devices has been described.[25] Future work developing and executing large systematic trials testing population health benefits for patients receiving care via increasingly connected health information systems is needed.

Although the study of system-based effects of wearables on health and cost outcomes remains embryonic, the proliferation of individual technologies for niche populations and specialties provides a broad indication of how devices are currently being used by consumers to assess elements of their health and by clinicians to enhance patient management. This article reviews the implementation of wearable devices across various specialties and medical education practices, with an emphasis on those technologies made available direct to consumers.

DIRECT TO CONSUMER

The most common direct-to-consumer wearable device is the smartphone. With an installation base numbering in the billions of devices, smartphones provide one of the most promising platforms for mobile health interventions, and software applications pledging to improve or track metrics of health are common and widely popular. From activity trackers that measure number of steps, calories burned, or hours sitting a day to telemedicine platforms that allow users to engage in video consultations for minor complaints, health-based apps promise easier weight loss, better sleep, and decreased primary care costs. However, a paucity of literature exists examining these claims outside the context of clinical research studies with additional interventions and protocols. It remains unclear whether outcomes or economics are significantly affected by the use of the consumer independent of clinical oversight or management.[26] Firmer evidence exists for using mobile devices as a means of measuring clinical parameters.

Cardiology

Remote monitoring of patient physiology has been a key tool in the management of many cardiac conditions. Portable technology for the recording of the ECG has existed for more than 70 years,[27] and modern Holter monitors are mainstays in the work-up of new-onset syncopal episodes or arrhythmias, although the relative bulk and obtrusiveness of monitoring devices raise concerns for patient satisfaction and compliance.[28] Modern consumer-wearable devices offer an opportunity to capture some of the clinically relevant information with improved form factors and expansive data storage and transmission capabilities.[29]

The accuracy of heart rate monitoring by commercially available wearables has been assessed, with heart rate measurement at a state of rest more reliable than during various modalities of exercise, although in each setting the photoplethysmography that measures the absorption of light during and after pulsations of blood through skin has been found to be uniformly less accurate than traditional electrophysiologic monitoring.[30] Implementation of specialized computer algorithms has been used to identify dysrhythmias. Tison and colleagues[31] described "teaching" a specialized computer "neural network" to identify variances in heart rate among nearly 10,000 patients enrolling in a remote cohort study consistent with the physiology of atrial fibrillation (AF), as measured by Apple Watch photoplethysmography. The Apple Watch heart rate–based detection method was also less sensitive and specific compared with standard 12-lead ECG. This effect is likely not clinically significant when assessing for basic dysrhythmias such as AF, but may lead to missed abnormalities or misdiagnosis of more subtle abnormalities.

Turakhia and colleagues[32] conducted a prospective study enrolling more than 400,000 patients using the Apple Watch device. In addition to monitoring for heart rate irregularities consistent with AF by way of a specialized pulse-detection algorithm, the study was designed to determine whether notifications from the device resulted in increased follow-up with medical providers and featured a specialized app developed for the Apple Watch that facilitated the enrollment of participants into the study. Once enrolled, patients detected to have multiple episodes of irregular heart rates were given a specialized alert that then engaged a video conference call with a study physician who conducted further history taking and determined whether the patients were eligible for the next step in the study, which entailed patients being mailed a single-channel ambulatory ECG detection device. Additional episodes of potential AF or other arrhythmias detected by both the pulse detection algorithm and ECG device resulted in study physicians recommending patients seek direct care with their primary providers. Findings presented at the American Cardiology Conference in 2019 noted that 0.5% of study participants received app-based notification of pulse irregularity, and that 34% of these patients later using the portable ECG monitor were found to have episodes of AF. Of the patients who were originally informed by the app of arrhythmias, 54% sought follow-up care with non-study medical providers.[33]

In addition to heart rate detection, handheld devices capable of recording ECGs have been described since the 1990s,[34] and several platforms harness the modern smartphones to facilitate ECG procurement, storage, and transmission. The Kardia-Mobile product line (AliveCor, San Francisco, CA) consists of specialized cases for a variety of smartphones and tablets that contain electrodes capable of obtaining a single-lead ECG.[35] The products have been cleared by the FDA for consumer use to record and monitor for basic dysrhythmias and have been used in studies screening for AF, prolonged corrected QT intervals, and pediatric tachyarrhythmias.[36–39] The arrival of built-in ECG functionality in the Apple Watch Series 4 may further increase the sensitivity of these devices for cardiac rhythm analysis, although, with only 2 electrodes providing a single lead, it is clear that the traditional 12-lead ECG will remain the gold standard of electrophysiologic analysis, at least for now.[40]

Bariatric Medicine

Weight management has been an attractive target for a variety of mobile applications, wearable devices, and digital consumer technologies. Multiple survey studies have shown that overweight and obese patients across different populations are open to the incorporation of activity trackers and smartphone apps into preexisting fitness and diet routines. Wang and colleagues[41] performed a small trial with 69 overweight and obese adults who were given FitBit One activity trackers to monitor daily exercise, with half the group randomized to additionally receive short message service (SMS) text messages promoting exercise via mobile phones. Participants were found to have marginal increases of less than 5 minutes in daily activity with the addition of activity trackers compared with their baseline, and no additional benefit was detected in the SMS group.[41] Jakicic and colleagues[42] conducted a larger randomized clinical trial with 471 subjects between the ages of 18 and 35 years with body mass indexes ranging from 25 to 40 and who were initially assigned specialized diets, exercise plans, and behavioral coaching with group counseling. Six months into the study, subjects gained access to a Web site with further weight loss information, specialized SMS messages, and phone-based counseling sessions. A randomized subset was then additionally given a wearable activity tracker interfacing with a Web-based application that gave feedback on exercise and allowed the logging of caloric intake. The subgroup with the wearable intervention had less weight loss than the comparable non-wearable group. A study by Finkelstein and colleagues[43] combining the use of activity trackers with cash or charitable donation exercise incentives was also unable to show any tangible health benefits from their use. The literature pertaining to the use of activity trackers and mobile applications for weight loss practices suggests that the utility may be optimized when designed to execute a previously constructed evidence-based program.[44]

Endocrinology

The effective management of diabetes mellitus (DM) requires significant effort and attention from patients to track, understand, and act on a vast range of data (ranging from blood glucose levels, to insulin dosing, to complex nutritional information). Competence with, and adherence to, therapeutic regimens has been associated with improved glycemic control. The potential of software and wearables to acquire and organize personal DM information has attracted interest in researchers seeking to enhance the ability of patients and clinicians to actively manage the condition.

An SMS-based diabetes support platform implemented in a large employer-based health plan in Chicago was associated with study participants reporting an increase in blood glucose monitoring, diabetic foot examinations, and diabetic medication compliance, with a subsequent decrease in hemoglobin A1c (HbA1c) measurements and number and cost of outpatient clinic appointments.[45] A proliferation of mobile applications focusing on diabetes and related concerns have accompanied the exponential increase in smartphone adoption and use, many of which target American Diabetes Association and American Association of Clinical Endocrinologists practice guidelines and standards of care for the management of diabetes.[46] An early randomized pilot study with patients with type II DM found that the use of a cell phone software program providing medication reminders, blood glucose tracking, and instructions for treatment of high or low blood glucose levels was associated with a larger decrease in HbA1c levels compared with the control group.[47] Larger, more recent studies indicate that widespread adoption of evidence-based glycemic control apps may provide similar sustained benefits across the health care ecosystem.[48,49]

DEVICES USED OR MANAGED BY CLINICIANS

In addition to direct-to-consumer technologies, wearable devices offer the potential to change how clinicians practice and manage patients in both the inpatient and outpatient settings. The following discussion focuses on devices used to improve access to consultant opinions, provide alternate procedural functionality, and facilitate organization of clinical and personal health data among several specialties.

Cardiology

In addition to electrophysiology, application of wearable devices in the interventional cardiology space has been described. Duong and colleagues[50] reported on the use of Google Glass as a telemedicine solution for the remote interpretation of coronary angiogram, and Opolski and colleagues[51] developed a virtual reality system displayed on a wearable computer that projected three-dimensional computed tomographic angiography of occluded coronary arteries to assist in percutaneous revascularization.

Dermatology

As with many medical subspecialties, uneven geographic distribution, a limited number of training positions, and an aging population have combined to create a shortage of dermatologists. Telemedicine has been proposed as a solution to rectify access disparities, and wearable devices may assist in facilitating remote care. Studies have described using the hands-free real-time video calling and image capture functionality of Google Glass to allow teleconference with dermatologists in the setting of micrographic surgery and allergy consultations.

Emergency Medicine

The use of wearables by emergency physicians has been well documented. Chai and colleagues[52] described using a version of the Google Glass for emergency department dermatology consultations, and several researchers have identified the portable, compact, and hands-free nature of the technology as being ideal for supporting first responders in disaster situations.[53]

Particular focus has been applied to Google Glass as a platform for teletoxicology evaluations. Chai and colleagues[54] additionally reported a series of 18 toxicology consultations conducted via Google Glass, with nearly 90% of the video calls featuring a high enough image resolution and minimal latency to facilitate clinical decision making. More than half of the consultations resulted in a change in management based on the transmitted information, with 6 patients receiving specific antidotes prescribed from findings obtained via Google Glass–facilitated examination.[54] Skolnik and colleagues[55] performed an expanded prospective observational cohort study with 50 patients that included the transmission of ECG data via Google Glass as well. Respondents found the technology largely reliable to perform remote examinations.

A study by Wu and colleagues[56] examined heads-up displays (HUDs) as a potential facilitator of ultrasonography-guided central venous cannulation by trainees. Real-time ultrasonography imaging displayed by Google Glass allowed participants to place central lines on a task trainer with the superimposed ultrasonography feed in direct vision. Wu and colleagues[56] hypothesized that limiting the need for the traditional turning to and from the ultrasonography machine to the procedure would minimize inadvertent hand movements during the procedure. Although the small sample size of 40 participants across different competence and learning levels did not produce significant results, the procedure was noted to take longer with Google Glass than with the traditional ultrasonography-guided technique.

Endocrinology

Regular self-monitoring of blood glucose levels remains a compliance challenge for clinicians treating diabetic patients, with nonadherence behaviors having complex psychosocial foundations. The need for repeated painful finger sticks with small lancet needles has led to the search for and development of alternate methods to assess glucose levels, and continuous glucose monitors (CGMs) offer such a solution. The prototypical CGM comprises a small sensor placed subcutaneously that measures glucose concentrations in the interstitial fluid. Although the glucose gradient between blood and interstitial fluid ensures a delay before reaching equilibrium that precludes real-time assessment of blood glucose levels for the purpose of prandial insulin bolus dosing, the data related to glucose trends over time have nevertheless contributed to advances in diabetes management, including the development of tools for prediction of hypoglycemic or hyperglycemic episodes. In the Daily Injections and Continuous Glucose Monitoring in Diabetes (DIAMOND) trial, Beck and colleagues[57] found that, in a group of 158 type 1 diabetic patients randomized to either CGM or traditional blood glucose checks for a 24-week period, the CGM group had a significantly greater decrease in HbA1c levels, a finding replicated in related studies. Work continues on novel wearable modalities for glucose sensing, with the popular news media focusing on Google's further development of research surrounding contact lenses that can measure glucose content in tears.[58]

One major challenge with CGM data is that the data sets are significantly larger than those from finger-stick glucometers, and providers have not traditionally had access to this information. Kumar and colleagues[20] described the first successful integration of CGM data in the EHR using a standard consumer interface from Apple, and subsequent studies have confirmed this approach as feasible and patient friendly.[59]

The combination of wearables with traditional medical devices, CGMs have recently been connected to subcutaneous insulin pumps, forming closed-loop systems in which algorithms working with glucose data received from CGMs are used to adjust the continuous delivery of insulin; in effect, functioning as rudimentary artificial pancreases.[60] Garg and colleagues[61] reported a multicenter study with 129 type 1 diabetics treated with a Medtronic-based closed-loop platform (Medtronic, Northridge, CA) for a 3-month period. Although patients still had to enter information related to carbohydrate loads and perform finger sticks to ensure safe bolus dosing, the platform was shown to be safe and effective at maintaining basal glucose levels, and subsequent studies have suggested that such systems may also contribute to improved glycemic control.

The potential benefits provided by this expanding collection of continuous glucose monitors, including novel noninvasive monitors, support apps, PHR integration, insight from population-based informatics, and even closed-loop insulin delivery systems, conjures an exciting future in which the management of this chronic condition becomes less arduous and expensive.

Neurology and Psychiatry

Investigators have suggested a broad array of use cases for quantifying the brain.[62] Patients with epilepsy disorders represent another population with an often difficult to manage chronic condition, with seizure frequency being particularly unpredictable and associated with significant potential morbidity.[63] The biometric data collected by wearables have been examined to determine whether early recognition of seizure activity can be measured. Detection of seizures through measurement of motion by accelerometry as detected by a commercially available smart watch was found to be significantly lacking in accuracy,[64] although algorithms generated from a combination of wearable motion and electrodermal data seem to be promising.[65]

Autism spectrum disorders (ASDs) are characterized in part by difficulties with socialization, including the processing of behavioral cues such as facial expressions. Supplementary visual information has long been recognized as a valuable tool to assist patients with ASDs in navigating intrapersonal interaction.[66] Work by The Autism Glass Project at Stanford Medicine has shown the potential utility of HUDs, including Google Glass, in providing a platform for therapeutic tools, including structured play, real-time visual cues, and monitoring of eye contact.[67] A recently published randomized clinical trial by the same group suggested that autistic patients using these technologies in conjunction with standard applied behavioral analysis treatment subsequently scored higher on certain behavioral indices compared with a control group receiving only the standard-of-care intervention.[68]

HUDs have additionally been evaluated as a telemedicine solution for neurorehabilitation and physical therapy purposes,[69] and interest has focused on using virtual reality systems such as the Oculus Rift as modalities for assisting patients dealing with acute and chronic pain in distracting and refocusing attention.[70]

Pain Management

The increasing prevalence of opioid use disorder in the United States is a public health crisis with a significant economic and societal cost in addition to the tens of thousands of lives lost every year. Innovative methods for helping to prospectively monitor patients at particular risk for adverse outcomes are in high demand, and multiple investigators have suggested that wearable devices may be of use in this context. Proof-of-concept work using biosensors similar in size and function to activity trackers that monitor temperature, movement, and electrical activity across the skin have developed physiologic profiles that are consistent with acute opioid use, although implementation of this technology as part of a monitoring or treatment program has, to our knowledge, not been described.[71]

Pulmonology and Sleep Medicine

Many commercially available smartphone applications and wearable devices feature functionality that claims to evaluate metrics of sleep quality. Evaluation by most hardware is accomplished by technology such as accelerometry that detects movement, with the device assessing low-movement periods as being consistent with sleep. Such technology is of limited utility in demarcating complex sleep behaviors or stages of sleep.[72] Software algorithms incorporating additional biometric data, including respiratory and heart rate variations, have been described,[73] and combined with wearable pulse oximetry sensors have been used in smartphone-based platforms to detect episodes of obstructive sleep apnea (OSA).[74] Surrel and colleagues[75] described an IoT OSA monitoring system using a single-lead ECG linked via Bluetooth to a smartphone, allowing continuous monitoring over a period of weeks. Despite advances, wearable sensors have not yet been able to replicate the reliability and granularity of data provided by polysomnography, the gold standard sleep medicine study.[76]

Surgery

HUDs have been widely investigated within the surgical subspecialties as platforms to facilitate remote consultation and assistance between surgeons and for providing enhanced or augmented visualization of relevant operative anatomy.[77] Microsoft's HoloLens has been the focus of proof-of-concept studies in neurologic surgery,[78] vascular surgery,[79] orthopedics,[80] and plastic surgery,[81] whereas Google Glass has been trialed in the pediatric surgery[82] and transplant surgery arenas,[83] among others.[84] The ophthalmology literature has reported on the use of modified HUDs as an alternate method of fundoscopy, providing a mobile and economical alternative to conventional hardware.[85] Virtual reality has long been recognized as a way to acquire task-based proficiency,[86] and work has continued to focus on the utility of HUDs displaying augmented or virtual reality environments as educational tools for surgical trainees.[87] In addition to facilitating direct learning, HUDs such as Google Glass have also been used by educators for the evaluation of trainees in simulation-based encounters.[88,89]

SUMMARY

The rapid proliferation of consumer-wearable devices, smartphone applications, and ancillary technology such as virtual and augmented reality form a key and increasingly important opportunity for modern health care. The potential of these tools to encourage engagement with clinicians, facilitate chronic disease management, and collect vast amounts of health data has long been touted, and the prospect of a future health care IoT ecosystem delivering personalized, high-quality care while decreasing cost burdens is a common vision. Especially promising are the synergies between wearables and other emerging technologies, such as artificial intelligence. The vast amounts of data collected by consumer devices may be particularly useful when analyzed by complex algorithms that may allow enhanced pattern recognition and clinical decision support, which is an increasingly important consideration in the setting of improved functionality. If wearable devices are to be relied on to provide early warning of disorder, it is attendant that appropriate information is conveyed to the patient to allow an escalation of care. Similar information may be provided in advance to clinicians to allow quicker triage and assignation of resources. To date, clinical decision support implications in the setting of wearable devices have not been widely studied.

Although there is no shortage of interesting clinical applications of these technologies, there remains a dearth of high-quality literature showing significant benefit to outcomes or other clinical metrics. The clearest advantages of these devices to date may lie in their ability to facilitate telemedicine applications to assist with significant geographic and socioeconomic disparities in access to care. Despite these caveats, with ever-increasing functionality, an increasing blurring of the lines between traditional implanted medical devices and wearables, and synergy with emerging informatics technologies, wearables promise to remain an area of active and exciting research and development.

DISCLOSURE

The authors have nothing to disclose.

REFERENCES

1. Richesson RL, Andrews JE, Hollis KF. Introduction to clinical research informatics. In: Richesson RL, Andrews JE, editors. Clinical research informatics. Cham (Switzerland): Springer International Publishing; 2019. p. 3–15. https://doi.org/10.1007/978-3-319-98779-8_1.

2. Longhurst CA, Pageler NM, Palma JP, et al. Early experiences of accredited clinical informatics fellowships. J Am Med Inform Assoc 2016;23(4):829–34.

3. Hawthorne KH, Richards L. Personal health records: a new type of electronic medical record. Rec Management J 2017;27(3):286–301.
4. Bassett DR, Freedson PS, John D. Wearable activity trackers in clinical research and practice. Kinesiol Rev (Champaign) 2019;8(1):11–5.
5. Iqbal MH, Aydin A, Brunckhorst O, et al. A review of wearable technology in medicine. J R Soc Med 2016;109(10):372–80.
6. Gubbi J, Buyya R, Marusic S, et al. Internet of Things (IoT): a vision, architectural elements, and future directions. Future Gener Comput Syst 2013;29(7):1645–60.
7. Fargen KM, Frei D, Fiorella D, et al. The FDA approval process for medical devices: an inherently flawed system or a valuable pathway for innovation? J Neurointerv Surg 2013;5(4):269–75.
8. Shuren J, Patel B, Gottlieb S. FDA regulation of mobile medical apps. JAMA 2018;320(4):337.
9. Teng XF, Zhang YT, Poon CCY, et al. Wearable medical systems for p-Health. IEEE Rev Biomed Eng 2008;1:62–74.
10. Van Hoof C, Penders J. Addressing the healthcare cost dilemma by managing health instead of managing illness - an opportunity for wearable wireless sensors. In: Design, automation & test in Europe conference & Exhibition (DATE), 2013. Grenoble (France): IEEE Conference Publications; 2013. p. 1537–9.
11. Poon CCY, Zhang YT. Perspectives on high technologies for low-cost healthcare. IEEE Eng Med Biol Mag 2008;27(5):42–7.
12. Milani RV, Lavie CJ. Health care 2020: reengineering health care delivery to combat chronic disease. Am J Med 2015;128(4):337–43.
13. Levine JA. The application of wearable technologies to improve healthcare in the World's Poorest People. TI 2017;08(02):83–95.
14. Holtz B, Vasold K, Cotten S, et al. Health care provider perceptions of consumer-grade devices and apps for tracking health: a pilot study. JMIR Mhealth Uhealth 2019;7(1):e9929.
15. Beaudin JS, Intille SS, Morris ME. To track or not to track: user reactions to concepts in longitudinal health monitoring. J Med Internet Res 2006;8(4):e29.
16. Bergmann JHM, McGregor AH. Body-worn sensor design: what do patients and clinicians want? Ann Biomed Eng 2011;39(9):2299–312.
17. Chang Y-J, Chen C-H, Lin L-F, et al. Wireless sensor networks for vital signs monitoring: application in a nursing home. Int J Distrib Sens Netw 2012;8(11):685107.
18. Xing F, Peng G, Liang T, et al. Challenges for deploying IoT wearable medical devices among the ageing population. In: Streitz N, Konomi S, editors. Distributed, ambient and pervasive interactions: understanding humans, Vol. 10921. Cham (Switzerland): Springer International Publishing; 2018. p. 286–95. https://doi.org/10.1007/978-3-319-91125-0_25.
19. Vuppalapati C, Ilapakurti A, Kedari S. The role of big data in creating sense EHR, an integrated approach to create next generation mobile sensor and wearable data driven Electronic Health Record (EHR). In: 2016 IEEE Second International Conference on Big Data Computing Service and Applications (BigDataService). Oxford, United Kingdom: IEEE; 2016. p. 293–296. doi:10.1109/BigDataService. March 29 - April 1 2016.
20. Kumar RB, Goren ND, Stark DE, et al. Automated integration of continuous glucose monitor data in the electronic health record using consumer technology. J Am Med Inform Assoc 2016;23(3):532–7.
21. Ryu B, Kim N, Heo E, et al. Impact of an electronic health record-integrated personal health record on patient participation in health care: development and

randomized controlled trial of MyHealthKeeper. J Med Internet Res 2017;19(12): e401.

22. Weenk M, van Goor H, Frietman B, et al. Continuous monitoring of vital signs using wearable devices on the general ward: pilot study. JMIR Mhealth Uhealth 2017;5(7):e91.

23. Joshi M, Ashrafian H, Aufegger L, et al. Wearable sensors to improve detection of patient deterioration. Expert Rev Med Devices 2019;16(2):145–54.

24. Dameff C, Clay B, Longhurst CA. Personal health records: more promising in the smartphone era? JAMA 2019;321(4):339.

25. Choi A, Shin H. Longitudinal healthcare data management platform of healthcare IoT devices for personalized services. J Univers Comput Sci 2018;24(9):1153–69.

26. DiFilippo KN, Huang W-H, Andrade JE, et al. The use of mobile apps to improve nutrition outcomes: a systematic literature review. J Telemed Telecare 2015;21(5): 243–53.

27. Holter NJ, Generelli JA. Remote recording of physiological data by radio. Rocky Mt Med J 1949;46(9):747–51.

28. Fensli R, Dale JG, O'Reilly P, et al. Towards improved healthcare performance: examining technological possibilities and patient satisfaction with wireless body area networks. J Med Syst 2010;34(4):767–75.

29. Pevnick JM, Birkeland K, Zimmer R, et al. Wearable technology for cardiology: an update and framework for the future. Trends Cardiovasc Med 2018;28(2):144–50.

30. Gillinov S, Etiwy M, Wang R, et al. Variable accuracy of wearable heart rate monitors during aerobic exercise. Med Sci Sports Exerc 2017;49(8):1697–703.

31. Tison GH, Sanchez JM, Ballinger B, et al. Passive detection of atrial fibrillation using a commercially available Smartwatch. JAMA Cardiol 2018;3(5):409.

32. Turakhia MP, Desai M, Hedlin H, et al. Rationale and design of a large-scale, app-based study to identify cardiac arrhythmias using a smartwatch: the apple heart study. Am Heart J 2019;207:66–75.

33. Apple heart study identifies AFib in small group of apple watch wearers. American College of Cardiology. Available at: https://www.acc.org/latest-in-cardiology/articles/2019/03/08/15/32/sat-9am-apple-heart-study-acc-2019. Accessed July 13, 2019.

34. Buntz B. Ahead of his time. MDDI Online. 2012. Available at: https://www.mddionline.com/ahead-his-time. Accessed July 13, 2019.

35. KardiaMobile. AliveCor, Inc. Available at: https://store.alivecor.com/products/kardiamobile. Accessed July 13, 2019.

36. Halcox JPJ, Wareham K, Cardew A, et al. Assessment of remote heart rhythm sampling using the alivecor heart monitor to screen for atrial fibrillation: the REHEARSE-AF study. Circulation 2017;136(19):1784–94.

37. Nguyen HH, Van Hare GF, Rudokas M, et al. SPEAR trial: smartphone pediatric ElectrocARdiogram trial. Hund T, ed. PLoS One 2015;10(8):e0136256.

38. Chung EH, Guise KD. QTC intervals can be assessed with the AliveCor heart monitor in patients on dofetilide for atrial fibrillation. J Electrocardiol 2015; 48(1):8–9.

39. Lau JK, Lowres N, Neubeck L, et al. iPhone ECG application for community screening to detect silent atrial fibrillation: a novel technology to prevent stroke. Int J Cardiol 2013;165(1):193–4.

40. Orellana VH. Apple Watch ECG vs. hospital EKG: not the results I was expecting. 2019. Accessed August 7, 2019. Available at: https://www.cnet.com/news/apple-watch-ecg-ekg-watchos-vs-hospital-medical-grade-detected-strange-heart-rhythm/.

41. Wang JB, Cadmus-Bertram LA, Natarajan L, et al. Wearable sensor/device (Fitbit One) and SMS text-messaging prompts to increase physical activity in overweight and obese adults: a randomized controlled trial. Telemed J E Health 2015;21(10):782–92.

42. Jakicic JM, Davis KK, Rogers RJ, et al. Effect of wearable technology combined with a lifestyle intervention on long-term weight loss: the IDEA randomized clinical trial. JAMA 2016;316(11):1161.

43. Finkelstein EA, Haaland BA, Bilger M, et al. Effectiveness of activity trackers with and without incentives to increase physical activity (TRIPPA): a randomised controlled trial. Lancet Diabetes Endocrinol 2016;4(12):983–95.

44. Breton ER, Fuemmeler BF, Abroms LC. Weight loss-there is an app for that! but does it adhere to evidence-informed practices? Transl Behav Med 2011;1(4): 523–9.

45. Nundy S, Dick JJ, Chou C-H, et al. Mobile phone diabetes project led to improved glycemic control and net savings for Chicago plan participants. Health Aff 2014;33(2):265–72.

46. Sieverdes JC, Treiber F, Jenkins C, et al. Improving diabetes management with mobile health technology. Am J Med Sci 2013;345(4):289–95.

47. Quinn CC, Clough SS, Minor JM, et al. WellDoc ^{TM} mobile diabetes management randomized controlled trial: change in clinical and behavioral outcomes and patient and physician satisfaction. Diabetes Technol Ther 2008;10(3):160–8.

48. Offringa R, Sheng T, Parks L, et al. Digital diabetes management application improves glycemic outcomes in people with type 1 and type 2 diabetes. J Diabetes Sci Technol 2018;12(3):701–8.

49. Hou C, Carter B, Hewitt J, et al. Do mobile phone applications improve glycemic control (HbA $_{1c}$) in the self-management of diabetes? A systematic review, meta-analysis, and GRADE of 14 randomized trials. Dia Care 2016;39(11):2089–95.

50. Duong T, Wosik J, Christakopoulos GE, et al. Interpretation of coronary angiograms recorded using google glass: a comparative analysis. J Invasive Cardiol 2015;27(10):443–6.

51. Opolski MP, Debski A, Borucki BA, et al. First-in-man computed tomography-guided percutaneous revascularization of coronary chronic total occlusion using a wearable computer: proof of concept. Can J Cardiol 2016;32(6):829.e11-13.

52. Chai PR, Wu RY, Ranney ML, et al. Feasibility and acceptability of google glass for emergency department dermatology consultations. JAMA Dermatol 2015; 151(7):794.

53. Cicero MX, Walsh B, Solad Y, et al. Do you see what I see? Insights from using google glass for disaster telemedicine triage. Prehosp Disaster Med 2015; 30(1):4–8.

54. Chai PR, Babu KM, Boyer EW. The feasibility and acceptability of google glass for teletoxicology consults. J Med Toxicol 2015;11(3):283–7.

55. Skolnik AB, Chai PR, Dameff C, et al. Teletoxicology: patient assessment using wearable audiovisual streaming technology. J Med Toxicol 2016;12(4):358–64.

56. Wu TS, Dameff CJ, Tully JL. Ultrasound-guided central venous access using google glass. J Emerg Med 2014;47(6):668–75.

57. Beck RW, Riddlesworth T, Ruedy K, et al. Effect of continuous glucose monitoring on glycemic control in adults with type 1 diabetes using insulin injections: the DIAMOND randomized clinical trial. JAMA 2017;317(4):371.

58. Badugu R, Lakowicz JR, Geddes CD. A glucose sensing contact lens: a non-invasive technique for continuous physiological glucose monitoring. J Fluoresc 2003;13(5):371–4.

59. Lewinski AA, Drake C, Shaw RJ, et al. Bridging the integration gap between patient-generated blood glucose data and electronic health records. J Am Med Inform Assoc 2019;26(7):667–72.
60. Trevitt S, Simpson S, Wood A. Artificial pancreas device systems for the closed-loop control of type 1 diabetes: what systems are in development? J Diabetes Sci Technol 2016;10(3):714–23.
61. Garg SK, Weinzimer SA, Tamborlane WV, et al. Glucose outcomes with the in-home use of a hybrid closed-loop insulin delivery system in adolescents and adults with type 1 diabetes. Diabetes Technol Ther 2017;19(3):155–63.
62. Stark DE, Kumar RB, Longhurst CA, et al. The quantified brain: a framework for mobile device-based assessment of behavior and neurological function. Appl Clin Inform 2016;7(2):290–8.
63. Bou Assi E, Nguyen DK, Rihana S, et al. Towards accurate prediction of epileptic seizures: a review. Biomed Signal Process Control 2017;34:144–57.
64. Patterson AL, Mudigoudar B, Fulton S, et al. SmartWatch by SmartMonitor: assessment of seizure detection efficacy for various seizure types in children, a large prospective single-center study. Pediatr Neurol 2015;53(4):309–11.
65. Poh M-Z, Loddenkemper T, Reinsberger C, et al. Convulsive seizure detection using a wrist-worn electrodermal activity and accelerometry biosensor: wrist-worn convulsive seizure detection. Epilepsia 2012;53(5):e93–7.
66. Quill KA. Visually cued instruction for children with autism and pervasive developmental disorders. Focus Autistic Behav 1995;10(3):10–20.
67. Washington P, Voss C, Haber N, et al. A wearable social interaction aid for children with autism. In: Proceedings of the 2016 CHI conference extended abstracts on human factors in computing systems - CHI EA '16. Santa Clara, CA: ACM Press; May 7 -12, 2016. p. 2348–2354. doi:10.1145/2851581.2892282.
68. Voss C, Schwartz J, Daniels J, et al. Effect of wearable digital intervention for improving socialization in children with autism spectrum disorder: a randomized clinical trial. JAMA Pediatr 2019;173(5):446.
69. De la Cruz F, Condori-Castillo E, Mauricio D, et al. Telemedicine model using smart glasses: a physical therapy rehabilitation study protocol. In: 2018 Congreso Internacional de Innovación y Tendencias En Ingeniería (CONIITI). Bogota, Colombia: IEEE; October 3- 5, 2018. p. 1–5. doi:10.1109/CONIITI.2018.8587106.
70. Hoffman HG, Meyer WJ, Ramirez M, et al. Feasibility of articulated arm mounted oculus rift virtual reality goggles for adjunctive pain control during occupational therapy in pediatric burn patients. Cyberpsychol Behav Soc Netw 2014;17(6):397–401.
71. Mahmud MS, Fang H, Wang H, et al. Automatic detection of opioid intake using wearable biosensor. In: 2018 International Conference on Computing, Networking and Communications (ICNC). Maui, HI: IEEE; March 5-8, 2018. p. 784–788. doi:10.1109/ICCNC.2018.8390334.
72. Poyares D, Hirotsu C, Tufik S. Fitness tracker to assess sleep: beyond the market. Sleep 2015;38(9):1351–2.
73. Cerutti S, Bianchi AM, Reiter H. Analysis of sleep and stress profiles from biomedical signal processing in wearable devices. In: 2006 International Conference of the IEEE Engineering in Medicine and Biology Society. New York: IEEE; August 31- September 3, 2006. p. 6530–6532. doi:10.1109/IEMBS.2006.260885.
74. Oliver N, Flores-Mangas F. HealthGear: a real-time wearable system for monitoring and analyzing physiological signals. In: International workshop on wearable and implantable body sensor networks (BSN'06). Cambridge, MA: IEEE; April 3-5, 2006. p. 61–64. doi:10.1109/BSN.2006.27.

75. Surrel G, Aminifar A, Rincon F, et al. Online obstructive sleep apnea detection on medical wearable sensors. IEEE Trans Biomed Circuits Syst 2018;12(4):762–73.
76. Mantua J, Gravel N, Spencer R. Reliability of sleep measures from four personal health monitoring devices compared to research-based actigraphy and polysomnography. Sensors 2016;16(5):646.
77. Shuhaiber JH. Augmented reality in surgery. Arch Surg 2004;139(2):170.
78. Incekara F, Smits M, Dirven C, et al. Clinical feasibility of a wearable mixed-reality device in neurosurgery. World Neurosurg 2018;118:e422–7.
79. Armstrong DG, Rankin TM, Giovinco NA, et al. A heads-up display for diabetic limb salvage surgery: a view through the google looking glass. J Diabetes Sci Technol 2014;8(5):951–6.
80. Condino S, Turini G, Parchi PD, et al. How to build a patient-specific hybrid simulator for orthopaedic open surgery: benefits and limits of mixed-reality using the Microsoft Hololens. J Healthc Eng 2018;2018:1–12.
81. Adabi K, Rudy H, Stern CS, et al. Abstract: optimizing measurements in plastic surgery through holograms with Microsoft Hololens. Plast Reconstr Surg Glob Open 2017;5:182–3.
82. Muensterer OJ, Lacher M, Zoeller C, et al. Google glass in pediatric surgery: an exploratory study. Int J Surg 2014;12(4):281–9.
83. Baldwin ACW, Mallidi HR, Baldwin JC, et al. Through the looking glass: real-time video using 'smart' technology provides enhanced intraoperative logistics. World J Surg 2016;40(1):242–4.
84. Wei NJ, Dougherty B, Myers A, et al. Using google glass in surgical settings: systematic review. JMIR Mhealth Uhealth 2018;6(3):e54.
85. Wang A, Christoff A, Guyton DL, et al. Google glass indirect ophthalmoscopy. JournalMTM 2015;4(1):15–9.
86. Seymour NE, Gallagher AG, Roman SA, et al. Virtual reality training improves operating room performance: results of a randomized, double-blinded study. Ann Surg 2002;236(4):458–63 [discussion: 463–4].
87. Dickey R, Srikishen N, Lipshultz L, et al. Augmented reality assisted surgery: a urologic training tool. Asian J Androl 2016;18(5):732.
88. Wu T, Dameff C, Tully J. Integrating Google Glass into simulation-based training: experiences and future directions. JBGC 2014;4(2):p49.
89. Tully J, Dameff C, Kaib S, et al. Recording Medical Students' encounters with standardized patients using google glass: providing end-of-life clinical education. Acad Med 2015;90(3):314–6.

Lessons Learned from Direct-to-Consumer Genetic Testing

Lauren M. Petersen, PhD, Joel A. Lefferts, PhD*

KEYWORDS

- Direct-to-consumer genetic testing • Cancer • *BRCA1* • *BRCA2*

KEY POINTS

- The direct-to-consumer genetic testing company 23andMe offers reports on carrier status for a select few pathogenic variants in the BRCA1/2 genes and the MUTYH gene that increase the risk of developing cancer.
- Direct-to-consumer genetic testing is often incomplete and the results can be misunderstood by individuals.
- Further studies are required to understand the appropriateness of population genetic testing without the direct oversight of a physician or genetic counselor.

HISTORY OF DIRECT-TO-CONSUMER TESTING

The introduction of next-generation sequencing technology and the completion of the human genome project in the early 2000s revolutionized the field of genomic research.[1,2] Looking to capitalize on the rapidly evolving field, a host of direct-to-consumer (DTC) testing companies emerged in the mid 2000s offering customers health-related genetic information without the need to involve a physician (**Fig. 1**). The first tests from companies such as 23andMe, Navigenics, and deCODEme were microarray-based genotyping assays that looked at single nucleotide polymorphisms (SNPs) in specific areas of the human genome. These tests cost around $1000 and offered such information as susceptibility to certain diseases based on specific genetic variants, although many of the claims made by these companies lacked scientific evidence. Although many DTC genetic testing companies received support in terms of capital investors, media coverage, and a broad customer base, these companies underwent increased scrutiny because they were not CLIA-certified laboratories and their tests were not clinically validated. State regulators and the US Food and Drug

[a] Department of Pathology and Laboratory Medicine, Dartmouth-Hitchcock Medical Center and Geisel School of Medicine at Dartmouth, One Medical Center Drive, Lebanon, NH 03756, USA
* Corresponding author.
E-mail address: Joel.A.Lefferts@hitchcock.org

Clin Lab Med 40 (2020) 83–92
https://doi.org/10.1016/j.cll.2019.11.005
0272-2712/20/© 2019 Elsevier Inc. All rights reserved.

labmed.theclinics.com

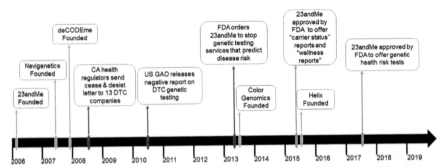

Fig. 1. Timeline of the major events in DTC genetic testing since 2006. CA, California; FDA, US Food and Drug Administration; GAO, Government Accountability Office.

Administration (FDA) have since introduced an increased number of regulations on many of the practices of DTC genetic companies. However, it remains unclear whether these companies should be allowed to offer clinically relevant testing. And, despite a multitude of controversies regarding the ethics and accuracies of such testing, DTC testing is a burgeoning business, with many new companies emerging each year offering panels on everything from cancer risk to information on phenotypic traits such as hair and eye color. Furthermore, the field is projected to continue growing at a rate of 25% annually, increasing from an estimated $684.7 million in 2017 to a projected $6.36 billion by 2028.[3]

The types of genetic tests being offered by DTC companies are numerous. The Association for Molecular Pathology (AMP) has classified the types of testing available from DTC companies into 4 distinct categories.[4] Ancestry testing is available for customers to gain insight into ethnic backgrounds and even connect with others who share common DNA markers. The second category designated by AMP consists of recreational tests that fall into the infotainment category. These tests do not provide health-related information, but instead report on such traits as eye color, hair thickness, and earlobe type. A third category of DTC genetic testing defined by AMP includes those related to business interests. These include wellness panels that predict muscle composition, deepness of sleep, and lactose intolerance. Although not clinically important, these types of tests often lead to third-party companies attempting to sell products (such as dietary supplements) or services based on the results of DTC genetic testing. The final category, designated as clinically meaningful by AMP, includes panels that provide information that can diagnose, predict, prognosticate, and/or reveal information relevant to an individual's health. Tests that fall under the clinically meaningful category include genetic testing for variants associated with cancer, diabetes, heart disease, and Parkinson's disease, as well as carrier screening tests that report the presence or absence of certain alleles linked to conditions, including cystic fibrosis, sickle cell anemia, and hereditary hearing loss. The clinically meaningful tests are surrounded by controversy for several reasons, including the following: (1) many tests are specific to certain types of populations (such as Ashkenazi Jews), (2) not every gene or genetic variant associated with a particular disease is evaluated, and (3) results may be misunderstood and/or misused by customers receiving results through the mail or over the Internet without an explanation provided by a medical professional.

Clinical guidelines indicate that certain kinds of genetic testing, in particular those that differ from routine carrier screening for pregnant women, are only appropriate for individuals suspected of having a genetic disease or whose family member has been formally diagnosed with one.[5,6] Yet now the general public has the option to order DTC disease-associated genetic testing regardless of how well they understand the analytical properties of the test, its limitations, and the potential implications of reported results for both themselves and family members. Consumers receive a kit in the mail, fill out a questionnaire, and send a saliva sample back to the company. Three to 5 weeks later, they receive results and, if customers opt in, can read reports that detail whether or not they have a variant associated with increased risk for a specific condition. Although the reports explicitly state that the results are not diagnostic and attempt to explain the limitations, including variant frequencies in different ethnic groups, there is no in-depth interpretation to ensure the customer fully understands the results. Ever since it became the first company to offer genetic testing to the general public, 23andMe has been at the forefront of the DTC testing industry. Its website, terms of service, and reports do highlight the limitations of its testing and urge consumers to consult with physicians before ordering the Genetic Health Risks and Carrier Status tests. However, physicians and genetic counselors have historically controlled health-related genetic testing by ordering, interpreting, and explaining results to patients so that proper steps, if needed, could take place under medical care.

Because of early concerns over DTC genetic testing there was an investigation in 2006 by the US Government Accountability Office.[7] Posing as customers, the US Government Accountability Office sent samples from the same individual to various laboratories and then compared results. Analysis of results from 4 companies found conflicting information regarding risk predictions for a number of diseases or conditions. For example, 1 donor was given reports that he was at below average, average, and above average risk for prostate cancer and hypertension from 3 separate companies. The US Government Accountability Office also asked experts to comment on claims made by different companies, including the accuracy of interpretive comments, and found a number of concerning and erroneous statements included in customers' results. Two companies claimed they were able to use customers' genetic information to predict athletic performance and the sport best suited to their future skill set. Additionally, 2 DTC companies were selling personalized supplements to customers that could cure disease, one going so far as claiming their supplement could repair damaged DNA, even though no there was no scientific basis for such claims. The final report outlined findings of deceptive marketing practices and misleading test results and, after congressional hearings, the FDA sent a letter to 23andMe ordering immediate discontinuation of their Personal Genome Service.[8] Other DTC genetic testing companies received similar letters. In response, 23andMe began validation studies to fulfill the FDA's regulatory review process, which included providing evidence that the public was capable of understanding the results. In 2015, 23andMe gained approval to offer carrier screening for hereditary Bloom syndrome. Two years later, in April of 2017, 23andMe received authorization to market genetic health risk tests for 10 conditions under their Personal Genome Service that included Parkinson's disease, Alzheimer's disease, and celiac disease. In March 2018, 23andMe received authorization from the FDA to test for 3 pathogenic variants in the *BRCA1* and *BRCA2* genes that confer increased risk for breast and ovarian cancers.

BRCA GENES AND BREAST AND OVARIAN CANCERS

The *BRCA* genes are involved in the cell's repair mechanism for DNA double-stand breaks, a pathway regulated by poly adenosine diphosphate-ribose polymerase.[9,10] A pathogenic mutation in either *BRCA1* or *BRCA2* leads to a decreased capacity to repair double strand breaks, which in turn can lead to accumulation of other mutations, resulting in a higher likelihood of developing cancer.[11–13] More than 1500 unique pathogenic variants that are linked to an increased risk of developing breast and ovarian cancer have been identified in *BRCA1* and more than 1700 similarly pathogenic variants identified in *BRCA2*.[14] Carriers of a *BRCA1/2* germline mutation have a 47% to 70% risk of developing breast cancer and a 10% to 50% chance of developing ovarian cancer by age 70.[6,15–17] Carriers are also at higher risk of other malignancies that include prostate, pancreatic, and gastrointestinal cancers. Studies have demonstrated the benefits of knowing one's *BRCA1/2* carrier status, because it often leads to increased screening and, if cancer is detected, it is usually at an earlier stage of disease with better prognosis.[6] Additionally, the knowledge of one's carrier status facilitates the use of targeted therapies; individuals with breast cancer and germline mutations in *BRCA1/2* have higher progression-free survival when treated with the poly adenosine diphosphate-ribose polymerase inhibitor talazoparib compared with individuals treated with standard therapies.[18] Cancer-free women with a family history and a pathogenic *BRCA1/2* variant have several options for decreasing their risk of developing breast or ovarian cancer. Prophylactic mastectomy results in up to a 97% reduced risk of developing breast cancer and increases overall survival.[6,19] Salpingo-oophorectomy decreases the risk of ovarian cancer by 80% to 90% in women between the ages of 40 and 45 years. Overall, the detection of a *BRCA1/2* mutation has serious and potentially life-altering implications.

Despite the importance of identifying germline *BRCA1/2* mutations, screening for the general population has not been deemed necessary. An in-depth review of clinical guidelines by Forbes and colleagues[20] compared 32 international guidelines for *BRCA1/2* testing, 11 of which were guidelines specific to the United States. Although not all US guidelines are in agreement, 5 of the 11 published guidelines, including the American College of Medical Genetics and Genomics and the National Society of Genetic Counselors, recommend genetic counseling before testing. Furthermore, the 11 US-based guidelines differ on their recommendations as to whether *BRCA* genetic screening is necessary even when individuals meet various criteria such as a familial or personal history of breast cancer. A number of guidelines from Canada and Europe also advise that testing should not occur at all unless appropriate genetic counseling is obtained first and emphasize that additional counseling following testing is important. As such, DTC companies offering *BRCA1/2* testing to any and all paying customers are not following clinical guidelines laid out by organizations such as the US National Comprehensive Cancer Network.

LIMITATIONS OF DIRECT-TO-CONSUMER GENETIC TESTING FOR *BRCA* VARIANTS

Although their chosen test methodology (genotyping by array) is capable of identifying only a specific subset of pathogenic variants, 23andMe's promotional material implies the capacity to detect all pathogenic variants. Genotyping by array works by detecting SNPs in a given sample. Although SNP arrays are powerful and thousands of SNPs can be assayed in 1 test, the variant of interest must be known beforehand. In general, SNP arrays only detect common variants and therefore not all SNPs for a given gene will be detected by this approach. The 23andMe *BRCA1/2* test highlights a common problem with using genotyping by array because it only detects 2 *BRCA1* pathogenic variants (5382insC and 185delAG) and only 1 *BRCA2* variant (617delT) out of the thousands of known mutations in these 2 genes. Furthermore, these 3 variants are found in an estimated 2% of people of Ashkenazi Jewish descent and 0% to 0.1% of the general population. Therefore, this test has little usefulness in patients of non-Ashkenazi Jewish heritage. Although 23andMe does include information in their

BRCA1/2 reports regarding the limited number of variants tested and the higher prevalence of the variants in individuals of Ashkenazi Jewish descent, negative results may still cause misunderstandings among customers regarding their risk of developing cancer. Individuals who receive negative results could be falsely reassured that they do not have a mutation in their *BRCA1/2* genes because the vast majority of pathogenic variants are not evaluated. For this reason, as well as a lack of clinical data supporting the use of general screening practices for cancer risk, medical professionals are uneasy about testing the general population for cancer predisposition genes such as *BRCA1/2*.

Furthermore, a negative result from 23andMe's *BRCA1/2* test does not eliminate the possibility of developing breast or ovarian cancer, and individuals should adhere to consensus screening guidelines, especially if there is family history. It should be noted that only 5% to 10% of breast cancer cases occur in individuals who carry a germline *BRCA1/2* mutation.[21] More than 50 hereditary cancer syndromes have been characterized and more than 100 genes have been identified that increase the risk of developing cancer.[22] However, environmental factors and lifestyle choices can also significantly influence the risk of developing cancer.[23]

Challenges Interpreting Direct-to-Consumer Genetic Test Results

A positive result from 23andMe's *BRCA1/2* test raises 4 important issues: (1) results are difficult to correctly interpret without the aid of a genetic counselor; (2) a positive result can induce stress about the chances of developing breast or ovarian cancer both in the individual who took the test as well as in family members; (3) there is a high reported rate of false positives in DTC genetic testing[24] and, therefore, confirmation testing is required; and (4) there is a need to consult with a primary care provider or genetic counselor after receiving a positive result. Although 23andMe encourages all customers to obtain medical support before and after their testing, it is unlikely most will seek counseling before ordering the testing. Marketing and promotions, such as the $70.00 off sale 23andMe had on Black Friday in 2018, further decrease the likelihood of individuals seeking medical care before ordering testing. Customers will receive their results over the Internet and may or may not be capable of understanding what a positive result means. An estimated 60% of customers use third-party tools to help them interpret and understand the results provided by companies, a clear indication that not enough information is being included on reports.[25] There is high potential for stress and anxiety for both the individual and in family members who may agonize over whether or not to get tested themselves. A study found that customers who received positive results from the *BRCA1/2* testing from 23andMe had the most anxiety about how it would impact their family, in particular their children.[26] The *BRCA1/2* and other Personal Genome Service test results are not meant to be diagnostic; however, this nuance is likely lost on most individuals who receive a positive result. Any positive result should be confirmed by a clinical diagnostic laboratory, a recommendation highlighted by a study by Ambry Genetics, which found that 40% of reported positive results from DTC genetic testing were false positives, including several cases where pathogenic variants were reported for *BRCA1/2* but were confirmed negative by sequencing at Ambry.[24] If a positive result is confirmed, long-term cancer risk-reducing steps should be discussed with a physician's oversight.[27] However, it has been reported that only approximately 30% of DTC genetic testing customers share the results with their doctor.[24,28] Further complicating matters is the fact that there are not enough genetic counselors to handle the huge increase in DTC genetic testing.[29] Collectively, this indicates that the health care community does not have the resources to properly accommodate patients with variants detected by DTC genetic testing, many of whom will require expensive follow-up. Owing to deviations from normal clinical guidelines governing genetic testing, it is highly unlikely that any confirmatory testing would be covered by insurance companies in these individuals.[30]

Genetic Testing of Minors

An additional issue is the use of DTC genetic testing for children. Guidelines from the American Academy of Pediatrics state in their policy that predictive genetic testing for adult-onset conditions should be deferred until the child is able to consent.[31] Yet if parents or guardians with to pursue genetic testing of a minor, those decisions should be made with clinical guidance. The American Medical Association's opinion is that genetic testing for children should only be performed under the care of a physician and with appropriate counseling when a child is at risk for a condition with established, effective prevention or treatment measures.[32] The American Medical Association also supports clinicians who refuse to pursue testing of a child when the parents request testing deemed to be unethical, and even to use legal means if necessary. DTC genetic companies allow parents to order any testing that is publicly available for their children, leading to potential concerns about positive results for a child who is unlikely to understand the results and, later in life, may not wish to have had the testing done in the first place. It can also lead to confusion and concerns for entire families, such as a case described by Moscarello and colleagues,[25] in which a 15 year-old girl was screened by DTC genetic testing and found to have a false-positive pathogenic variant in the *PKP2* gene. This variant was known to have a role in arrhythmogenic right ventricular cardiomyopathy. That result, along with an erroneous interpretation of a cardiac MRI test, led to the placement of an implanted cardioverter defibrillator. Once confirmatory genetic testing found that there was no variant in the *PKP2* gene and the cardiac MRI was normal, the device was taken out. Although this type of case is rare, it underscores the need for DTC companies to take into consideration that their results can have profound negative effects on customers, including those who have not directly consented to having such testing done.

Patient Privacy

Another (often poorly understood) concern for individuals who undergo DTC genetic testing is how companies handle their personal data and how exactly they protect customers' information. The commercialization of DNA sequencing introduces sensitive privacy issues because it reveals personal information about disease susceptibility, traits, and predispositions for both the individual and blood relatives. Furthermore, DTC genetic testing companies do not fall under the genetic privacy acts like the Health Insurance Portability and Accountability Act. As an example, 23andMe has a 25-page terms of service and a 29-page privacy statement that explains the company's sample handling practices, account set up, and the use of third parties.[33] Essentially, 23andMe reserves the right to use and share customers' data (even after customers delete their account) with partners to improve their services as long as the individual "cannot be reasonably identified." If participants choose to have their information included in research, they must sign a separate consent that also allows the company to share both personal and genetic information with third-party collaborators. Although 23andMe makes it clear that data will not be stored in public databases, it has already been reported that the company has sold de-identified information to pharmaceutical companies who are developing medical treatments.[27] At this time, regulations for genetic privacy are lacking.[34] More comprehensive security measures are necessary to address genetic data anonymization and misuse by DTC genetic companies.

POTENTIAL BENEFITS OF DIRECT-TO-CONSUMER GENETIC TESTING

Despite the many limitations described in this article, DTC genetic testing for *BRCA1/2* can be of benefit. Although more studies need to be conducted, the data collected thus far describing consumers' response to DTC genetic testing are reassuring. Customers with negative DTC genetic test results for *BRCA1/2* mutations have reported that they understand the results do not mean they are at lower risk of developing cancer and have not reported inappropriate actions such as ignoring recommended cancer screening.[26] Furthermore, many customers in whom *BRCA1/2* pathogenic variants were detected found the knowledge to be of benefit because it allows carriers to seek genetic counseling and better understand how to reduce their risk and that of family members.

To date, 23andMe reports having more than 10,000,000 customers and claims that more than 80% of customers have agreed to make their data available for research.[35] From a research perspective, access to data from so many individuals has the potential to make a significant impact in the progress of understanding a number of genetically related diseases. The 23andMe Research Team has been involved in a variety of different peer-reviewed publications that include genetic determinants to predict the age of Parkinson's disease onset, the genetics of asthma, and common risk variants linked to autism.[36–38] So long as participants in 23andMe's research projects understand what they are consenting to, the sheer numbers opting in creates a powerful approach to scientific discovery that most likely will have a positive impact on precision medicine in the near future.

ALTERNATE APPROACHES TO DIRECT-TO-CONSUMER GENETIC TESTING

Other DTC companies have taken slightly different approaches to genetic testing both in their methodologies and general practices of clinician involvement. Helix is an Illumina spin-off that performs a combination of microarray testing and whole exome sequencing. Exome sequencing is an unbiased approach that sequences all of the protein-coding regions in the human genome. In contrast with genotyping by array, exome sequencing has the ability to detect all mutations in protein-encoding genes, not just those included in a limited, predesigned array format. However, a limitation of exome sequencing is that the roles of most SNPs in the human genome are not completely understood, resulting in uninterpretable information. That said, Helix partners with companies such as PerkinElmer Genomics, the Mayo Clinic, and EverlyWell to report on risk assessment for certain cancers, the association of genetics and overall health, and food sensitivities, respectively. With consent, Helix can store customers' data to allow them to "sequence once, query often" so they can purchase access to more of their own genomic information without having to send in additional samples. Importantly, when an individual wants to order a test, Helix has an independent physician review the indications for testing on some of their DNA Products (without specifically explaining which tests specifically on their terms of service) to ensure the testing is appropriate. However, they do not directly provide a health care professional for counseling and only recommend that their customers consult a genetic counselor if they have specific questions interpreting their results. Another company, Color Genomics, that offers panels for hereditary cancer, heart disease, and pharmacogenomics testing to predict response to specific medications, has also chosen to include direct physician involvement for genetic testing. If a customer requests a test, a Color staff physician can order it or the customer can choose to order it through their own provider. Similar to Helix, Color Genomics also uses exome sequencing.

FUTURE CHALLENGES

There is a pressing need to improve the accuracy of DTC genetic testing, develop more effective ways of communicating test results, and ensure that participants fully understand reported results and take appropriate follow-up steps. If no regulatory changes are made, it is likely that companies will keep adding testing for more genes and diseases. As an example, 23andMe recently added a new Genetic Health Risk report that includes 2 genetic variants in the *MUTYH* gene (Y179C and G396D) that are associated with the hereditary colorectal cancer syndrome *MUTYH*-associated polyposis. As with their *BRCA1/2* test, the *MUTYH* testing is most applicable for a specific population, in this case people of Northern European descent.[39] Also echoing the *BRCA1/2* test is that more than 100 other variants have been linked to *MUTYH*-associated polyposis, making this another example of an incomplete analysis of a gene and its associated disease. If future studies uncover misuse of data or determine DTC genetic testing leads to harm, then the FDA may have to reconsider whether population-based DTC genetic testing should be allowed to continue without additional regulations.

SUMMARY

The question of whether the general population should be screened for cancer-associated germline mutations touches on several complex issues, including who should get tested, what genes should be evaluated, how pathogenic variants should be detected (ie, full gene sequencing, hotspot sequencing or allele-specific genotyping), and if there is any clinical usefulness to having such knowledge. Actions can be taken in individuals with positive *BRCA1/2* mutation status but there are few, if any, risk-reducing options for other cancer predisposition genes. How far should companies go to ensure customers can correctly interpret their genetic results? Should genetic testing for disease and cancer risks even be taking place outside a doctor's office? An additional set of questions faces companies who offer exome sequencing, including how much information to report: should all variants, including variants of unknown significance, be reported or just ones that have been proven to cause disease? Whose responsibility is it to provide updated reports once variants of uncertain significance become reclassified as likely pathogenic variants? Comprehensive answers to these questions require long-term follow-up with DTC genetic testing customers to understand the impact of the general population collecting their own genetic data. In the end, stricter regulations may be required to ensure the benefits of DTC genetic testing outweigh the risks.

ACKNOWLEDGMENTS

The authors thank Stephen Paige for his input and review of the article.

DISCLOSURE

The authors have nothing to disclose.

REFERENCES

1. Collins FS, Morgan M, Patrinos A. The Human Genome Project: lessons from large-scale biology. Science 2003;300(5617):286–90.
2. Shendure J, Ji H. Next-generation DNA sequencing. Nat Biotechnol 2008;26(10):1135–45.
3. Yang YT, Zettler PJ. Food and Drug Administration's regulatory shift on direct-to-consumer genetic tests for cancer risk. Cancer 2019;125(1):12–4.
4. Association for Molecular Pathology. Association for Molecular Pathology position statement: consumer genomic testing - June 2019. Available at: https://www.amp.org/AMP/assets/File/position-statements/2019/AMP_Position_Statement_Consumer_Genomics_FINAL.pdf. Accessed July 29, 2019.
5. Foulkes WD, Knoppers BM, Turnbull C. Population genetic testing for cancer susceptibility: founder mutations to genomes. Nat Rev Clin Oncol 2016;13(1):41–54.
6. Bayraktar S, Arun B. BRCA mutation genetic testing implications in the United States. Breast 2016;31:224–32.
7. Kutz GD. Direct-to-Consumer genetic tests: misleading test results are further complicated by deceptive marketing and other questionable practices. Available at: https://www.gao.gov/assets/130/125079.pdf. Accessed July 15, 2019.
8. Yim S-H, Chung Y-J. Reflections on the US FDA's warning on direct-to-consumer genetic testing. Genomics Inform 2014;12(4):151–5.
9. Khanna KK, Jackson SP. DNA double-strand breaks: signaling, repair and the cancer connection. Nat Genet 2001;27:247–54.
10. Shrivastav M, De Haro LP, Nickoloff JA. Regulation of DNA double-strand break repair pathway choice. Cell Res 2008;18:134–47.
11. Helleday T. The underlying mechanism for the PARP and BRCA synthetic lethality: clearing up the misunderstandings. Mol Oncol 2011;5(4):387–93.
12. Javle M, Curtin NJ. The potential for poly (ADP-ribose) polymerase inhibitors in cancer therapy. Ther Adv Med Oncol 2011;3(6):257–67.
13. Konishi H, Mohseni M, Tamaki A, et al. Mutation of a single allele of the cancer susceptibility gene BRCA1 leads to genomic instability in human breast epithelial cells. Proc Natl Acad Sci U S A 2011;108(43):17773–8.
14. Rebbeck TR, Friebel TM, Friedman E, et al. Mutational spectrum in a worldwide study of 29,700 families with BRCA1 or BRCA2 mutations. Hum Mutat 2018;39(5):593–620.
15. Gill J, Obley AJ, Prasad V. Direct-to-consumer genetic testing the implications of the US FDA's first marketing authorization for BRCA mutation testing. JAMA 2018;319(23):2377–8.
16. Lippi G, Mattiuzzi C, Montagnana M. BRCA population screening for predicting breast cancer: for or against? Ann Transl Med 2017;5(13):275.
17. Neff RT, Senter L, Salani R. BRCA mutation in ovarian cancer: testing, implications and treatment considerations. Ther Adv Med Oncol 2017;9(8):519–31.
18. Litton JK, Rugo HS, Ettl J, et al. Talazoparib in patients with advanced breast cancer and a germline BRCA mutation. N Engl J Med 2018;379(8):753–63.
19. Hartmann LC, Lindor NM. The role of risk-reducing surgery in hereditary breast and ovarian cancer. N Engl J Med 2016;374(5):454–68.
20. Forbes C, Fayter D, de Kock S, et al. A systematic review of international guidelines and recommendations for the genetic screening, diagnosis, genetic counseling, and treatment of BRCA-mutated breast cancer. Cancer Manag Res 2019;11:2321–37.

21. Febbraro T, Robison K, Wilbur JS, et al. Adherence patterns to National Comprehensive Cancer Network (NCCN) guidelines for referral to cancer genetic professionals. Gynecol Oncol 2015;138(1):109–14.

22. Rahman N. Realizing the promise of cancer predisposition genes. Nature 2014; 505(7483):302–8.

23. Stewart BW. Priorities for cancer prevention: lifestyle choices versus unavoidable exposures. Lancet Oncol 2012;13(3):e126–33.

24. Tandy-Connor S, Guiltinan J, Krempely K, et al. False-positive results released by direct-to-consumer genetic tests highlight the importance of clinical confirmation testing for appropriate patient care. Genet Med 2018;20(12):1515–21.

25. Moscarello T, Murray B, Reuter CM, et al. Direct-to-consumer raw genetic data and third-party interpretation services: more burden than bargain? Genet Med 2019;21(3):539–41.

26. Francke U, Dijamco C, Kiefer AK, et al. Dealing with the unexpected: consumer responses to direct-access BRCA mutation testing. PeerJ 2013;1:e8.

27. Artin MG, Stiles D, Kiryluk K, et al. Cases in precision medicine: when patients present with direct-to-consumer genetic test results. Ann Intern Med 2019; 170(9):643–51.

28. Bloss CS, Wineinger NE, Darst BF, et al. Impact of direct-to-consumer genomic testing at long term follow-up. J Med Genet 2013;50:393–400.

29. Ramos E, Weissman SM. The dawn of consumer-directed testing. Am J Med Genet C Semin Med Genet 2018;178(1):89–97.

30. Holland CMA, Arbe-Barnes EH, McGivern EJ, et al. The 10th Oxbridge varsity medical ethics debate-should we fear the rise of direct-to-consumer genetic testing? Philos Ethics Humanit Med 2018;13(1):14.

31. Hardart GE, Chung WK. Genetic testing of children for diseases that have onset in adulthood: the limits of family interests. Pediatrics 2014;134:S104–10.

32. Association AM. Genetic testing of children. Available at: https://www.ama-assn.org/delivering-care/ethics/genetic-testing-children. Accessed September 23, 2019.

33. 23andMe. Privacy policy. Available at: https://www.23andme.com/about/privacy. Accessed July 15, 2019.

34. Li J. Genetic information privacy in the age of data-driven medicine. IEEE Int Congr Big Data 2016;45:299–306.

35. 23andMe. About Us. Available at: https://mediacenter.23andme.com/company/about-us/. Accessed July 15, 2019.

36. Blauwendraat C, Heilbron K, Vallerga CL, et al. Parkinson's disease age at onset genome-wide association study: defining heritability, genetic loci, and α-synuclein mechanisms. Mov Disord 2019;34(6):866–75.

37. Grove J, Ripke S, Als TD, et al. Identification of common genetic risk variants for autism spectrum disorder. Nat Genet 2019;51(3):431–44.

38. Ferreira MAR, Mathur R, Vonk JM, et al. Genetic architectures of childhood- and adult-onset asthma are partly distinct. Am J Hum Genet 2019;104(4):665–84.

39. 23andMe. 23andMe's new MUTYH-associated polyposis report Looks at risk for hereditary colorectal cancer associated with MUTYH variants. Available at: https://blog.23andme.com/health-traits/23andmes-new-mutyh-report/. Accessed July 15, 2019.

The Ethics of Direct-to-Consumer Testing

Ann M. Gronowski, PhD*, Melissa M. Budelier, PhD

KEYWORDS

- Ethics • Direct to consumer testing • Direct access testing

KEY POINTS

- The core principles of biomedical ethics include: Respect for autonomy, beneficence, nonmaleficence, and justice.
- Direct to consumer laboratory testing is a rapidly growing sector of health care; however, there are many questions regarding the ethics of allowing consumers to order their own laboratory tests.
- Direct to consumer laboratory testing has the potential to increase patient autonomy and improve access to health care for certain patient populations.
- The conditions necessary for autonomy are not always met with direct to consumer laboratory testing and there are concerns that unnecessary testing by consumers leads to false-positive results and increased costs to the health care system.
- There is little research documenting the positive or negative effects of direct to consumer testing.

INTRODUCTION

The origins of direct to consumer (DTC) testing are undoubtedly rooted in the development of over-the-counter (OTC) tests that enable patients to perform their own biochemical measurements. Early examples of OTC tests include fingerstick glucose for diabetics and urine human chorionic gonadotropin to detect pregnancy. The first home pregnancy test was marketed in the late 1970s and, although now it is a well-accepted member of the DTC health care market, its introduction was fraught with ethical controversy. Although home pregnancy testing imparted privacy and autonomy to women, health professionals were concerned that home testing may cause harm because women would not properly perform the tests or they might become hysterical over their results.[1–3] Similar ethical concerns were raised 40 years later, when the first home human immunodeficiency virus testing device entered the market.[4] Both types of testing have safely been in place for many years without evidence

Department of Pathology and Immunology, Washington University School of Medicine, Box 8118, 660 South Euclid, St Louis, MO 63110, USA
* Corresponding author.
E-mail address: gronowski@wustl.edu

Clin Lab Med 40 (2020) 93–103
https://doi.org/10.1016/j.cll.2019.11.001
0272-2712/20/© 2019 Elsevier Inc. All rights reserved.

of harming consumers and the menu of OTC tests has grown considerably to include tests for ovulation, drug and alcohol use, and urinary tract infections.

Laboratory performed DTC testing first appeared in the early 1990s with companies such as Any Lab Test Now and Home Access Health offering a wide variety of tests directly to consumers. A 2016, a *Wall Street Journal* survey indicated that 76% of people surveyed thought that they should have the right to have their blood tested any time they want without a doctor's order.[5] Eighty percent of responders felt that results should go directly to the patient or both the patient and the doctor, and 91% thought that health insurance should reimburse for DTC blood tests that were used for both detection of illness and wellness monitoring.[5] Laws about who can order tests, what tests can be ordered, and whether a physician is needed as an intermediary vary state by state, but clearly consumers want more control of their health care. As a result, the DTC test market continues to grow rapidly and is expected to exceed $350 million by 2020.[6] Other articles in this special issue have covered the pros and cons of DTC testing. Here, we focus specifically on the ethical implications of DTC testing.

To understand the ethical implications of DTC testing, one needs to understand the fundamental concepts of biomedical ethics. The terms medical ethics and biomedical ethics are often used interchangeably and can be defined as "a system of moral principles that apply values to the practice of clinical medicine and in scientific research."[7] Modern biomedical ethics grew largely out of grossly unethical behavior, such as the heinous research studies conducted in Europe during World War II (which resulted in the Nuremburg Code, the Declaration of Geneva, and eventually the Declaration of Helsinki) as well as the Tuskegee Syphilis study conducted in the United States (which resulted in the Belmont Report).[8] The core principles of biomedical ethics include respect for autonomy, beneficence (doing good), nonmaleficence (avoiding harm), and justice (**Table 1**).[9]

Ethics and cultural morals are interconnected and vary between different cultures. Therefore, ethical issues can be difficult to resolve because solutions are relative to the values of the parties involved. Within hospitals, there are teams such as human studies review boards, ethics committees, and risk management that can help to discuss and resolve difficult ethical cases. In contrast, there are no bodies that specifically oversee DTC testing. As a result, there is limited regulation or oversight of which tests can be offered by DTC companies and how companies should help consumers to interpret their testing. This information contributes to the ethical debate.

Table 1	
Core principles of biomedical ethics	
Principle	Definition
Respect for autonomy	People are treated with respect and dignity. The autonomy of the person is maintained and persons are not deceived in any way. Autonomous decisions are respected and supported. People with diminished autonomy are entitled to protection.
Beneficence	A group of norms pertaining to relieving, lessening, or preventing harm and providing and balancing benefits against risks and costs.
Nonmaleficence	Avoiding the causation of harm.
Justice	The duty or obligation to treat people equally and to distribute, by allocating fairly, what is rightly due in terms of benefits, risks and cost.

In light of the unique challenges of DTC testing and the fundamental concepts of biomedical ethics, we will discuss the fundamental question, "Is it ethical to allow consumers to order their own laboratory testing?"

AUTONOMY

Certainly, one of the principal advantages of DTC testing is the autonomy that it can provide to consumers. The ability for consumers to order their own laboratory testing, without the aid of a physician or other health care professional, allows them to take ownership of their health care and increase their health care literacy. Advocates of DTC testing promote the concept that people have the right to know about certain aspects of their health, even if it is just out of curiosity. They also have the right to know about diseases they may have for which there is no cure, if they choose to know. In its most simple form, one could argue that autonomy is upheld by DTC testing. However, Beauchamp and Childress[9] describe 3 conditions that must be met to achieve autonomy, namely, intentionality, understanding, and noncontrol.

Intentional means that the action is planned and is not accidental. DTC testing, when ordered by an individual for that individual, would meet the criteria of intentional. The testing is selected and ordered, the consumer submits a sample of his or her own free will, and pays for the testing to be performed. However, the nature of DTC testing allows for surreptitious testing such as parents testing children by sending saliva for genetic analysis. In these cases, the child's autonomy is not maintained. The American Academy of Pediatrics and the American College of Medical Genetics strongly discourage the DTC genetic testing of children.[10]

The second condition of autonomy, according to Beauchamp and Childress,[9] is *understanding*. An action is not autonomous if the individual does not adequately understand it. Many of the arguments against DTC testing rest on the idea that consumers do not understand what they are ordering or the usefulness of the results. For some tests, the importance and usefulness may be easy for consumers to understand, for example, glucose or cholesterol testing. Other DTC tests have questionable usefulness, such as the $399.00 Cellular Nutritional Health (Micronutrient Test) offered by Any Lab Test Now (https://www.anylabtestnow.com/tests/cellular-nutritional-health/) which claims to measures the body's ability to "absorb 32 vitamins, minerals, antioxidants and other essential nutrients into white blood cells." The results can help to "reduce the risk of illness and disease related to such deficiencies." Do consumers understand the limited usefulness of such tests? Likewise, DTC companies provide access to genetic testing often without genetic counseling.[11] The type of genetic testing that is, performed (eg, single nucleotide polymorphism vs whole genome sequencing) can impact the predictive value of the results.[12] Is this factor understood by patients? Without genetic counseling, do consumers understand the potential consequences of the genetic test results on themselves and their family members?[13,14] Many physicians confess that even they themselves do not fully understand genetic testing.[13,14] In fact, in 2010, the US Government Accountability Office concluded that many DTC genetic tests were misleading and of no practical use.[15]

The third condition of autonomy is *noncontrol*. In other words, people should be free of controls that rob them of self-directedness.[9] There is concern that some DTC genetic testing companies have advertising that is misleading and exaggerates risk.[16] In the mid-2000s, Myriad Genetics was criticized for their DTC advertising campaign that exploited public anxiety about breast cancer and misled consumers into believing that all women should have expensive BRCA genetic testing. Mutations in BRCA genes are rare, and unless an individual is at an increased risk, testing is unnecessary and unlikely to be clinically useful.[17] Schaper and Schicktanz[18] reviewed various DTC genetic web sites and concluded that many contain persuasive messaging. They observed 3 aspects of DTC advertising: "(1) the use of material suggesting medical professional legitimacy as a trust-enabling tool, (2) the suggestion of empowerment as a benefit of using DTC genetic testing services, and (3) the narrative of responsibility as a persuasive appeal to a moral self-conception."[18]

DTC testing does provide the opportunity for autonomy. If consumers are not subject to false advertising, and if they order tests that they fully understand, for themselves, then autonomy is maintained. Autonomy is lost if any of these conditions fail to be met (**Table 2**).

BENEFICENCE

Does DTC testing provide benefit to consumers? There are remarkably few data on the benefits of DTC testing. Interestingly, the same is true of OTC and point-of-care testing. For instance, although we assume that OTC pregnancy tests allow consumers to identify pregnancy earlier and modify behavior, such as decreasing alcohol consumption and beginning prenatal vitamins, there are no data to support that this actually happens. Likewise, we assume point-of-care human chorionic gonadotropin testing in the emergency department decreases turnaround time, but there are no data to support this assumption. The same is true for DTC testing. DTC testing

Table 2 Ways in which DTC does and does not uphold the core ethical principles		
Core Ethical Principle	**Upheld**	**Not Upheld**
Autonomy	Consumers have the freedom to order tests on themselves with no health care professional. Promotes health care literacy and right to know.	Autonomy not upheld if lacking any of these: Intentionality (tests ordered on others such as children) Understanding (consumers are not knowledgeable about the usefulness or interpretation of test results) Noncontrol (consumers are attracted to DTC testing via false advertising)
Beneficence	Allows for easy monitoring of disease Allows for early diagnosis of disease	Little evidence that DTC testing improves heath
Nonmaleficence	Little evidence that DTC testing harms consumers	False positives leading to: Potential for inaccurate diagnosis Increased health care costs Unclear implications on privacy Accuracy concerns owing to a lack of oversight
Justice	Access to health care for low-income or uninsured individuals	Perceived risk of discrimination from vulnerable populations Expensive tests (such as genetic testing) may increase health care disparities

does serve as a bridge between physicians and patients and allows consumers to monitor existing medical conditions such as diabetes, cardiovascular disease risk factors, and disorders involving the thyroid, liver, and kidneys. Although performed in a DTC setting instead of a hospital or doctor's office, this testing is sometimes ordered at the direction of a physician. DTC testing also allows consumers to screen for medical conditions described elsewhere in this article earlier than might be possible if such testing required an appointment with a physician. Advocates suggest that this factor is especially important for people without health insurance who may avoid hospitals and clinics. Testing without a doctor's visit can save time and money and help patients to determine if they need to seek costly medical care. Also, the privacy afforded by DTC testing is attractive for people testing for certain conditions such as pregnancy or infectious diseases.

Giovanni and colleagues[19] conducted a survey of genetic counselors and medical geneticists asking about their experience with patients referred to them after DTC genetic testing. Their survey resulted in 133 responses describing 22 cases of clinical interactions. Most of the consultations (59%) were self-referred to the genetic professionals, but 32% were physician referred. Interestingly, 53% of the responders reported that the DTC genetic testing was clinically useful. BRCA1/2 testing was considered clinically useful in 86% of cases and 36% of other tests were also considered clinically useful.[19] However, even the authors state that further study is required to understand why BRCA1/2 testing was disproportionately (6/7 cases) associated with an impression of clinical usefulness. In addition, they reported that the estimated costs associated from their referrals ranged from very little to a high of $20,604, raising questions about the impact of DTC testing on the health care system. If the genetic testing was clinically useful, as they reported, then it could be argued that these dollars were well-spent.

In short, there are few published data to support or refute the benefit of DTC testing, whether it is physician or consumer directed. A lack of evidence is not a reason to discontinue DTC testing, but clearly more research with outcomes data is needed in this area.

NONMALEFICENCE

Can consumers be harmed by ordering their own laboratory tests? Much of the ethical debate regarding DTC testing is centered on this topic. Opponents argue that DTC testing causes harm to both individuals and society as a whole (through increased cost of health care). However, there is little evidence to support this claim.

False-Positive Results

Reference intervals for many (not all) tests are based on the central 95% of results from a normal population. By definition, 5% of the normal population falls outside this reference interval. Health care professionals are aware that laboratory tests should be chosen carefully, taking into account pretest probability, to minimize false positives. The more tests performed on patients, especially with a low pretest probability, the greater chance of generating a false-positive test result. Therefore, opponents of DTC testing argue that it is unethical for consumers to order DTC testing because they will order unnecessary tests and thereby increase the risk of harm from false-positive results. This argument against DTC testing assumes a degree of ignorance on the part of consumers and that they are ordering multiple unnecessary laboratory tests. However, there is no evidence to support this assumption. First, some DTC laboratory testing is actually performed at the direction of a physician to monitor existing conditions but the percentage of total DTC testing ordered by a physician is unknown. Many consumers seek DTC testing rather than clinical laboratory testing because it is convenient and the cost is transparent. Because DTC testing is generally not covered by insurance, it seems likely that consumers are choosing to pay for laboratory tests based on a specific concern and are not just ordering tests randomly. Also, not all reference intervals are derived from the central 95%. Cholesterol, for instance, is based on outcome studies and, hence, the 5% false-positive argument does not hold true for all tests.

Some of the concern over DTC laboratory test ordering could be alleviated by restricting DTC testing to a menu of tests that have well-defined clinical usefulness. An on-line search of DTC laboratories shows that consumers can order many tests that health care professionals would argue have very limited usefulness. Lovett and colleagues[20] conducted a study that examined DTC screening tests offered online. They found that virtually all the tests offered were not recommended by the US Preventive Services Task Force, or other specialty guidelines, for use as screening tests, suggesting that the tests had limited value and could lead to inaccurate diagnoses. However, the study contained no outcome data to suggest actual harm to patients. It should also be noted that this study included many companies that provide DTC radiologic screening tests, not just laboratory testing.

Concern has also been raised about the accuracy of some DTC genetic tests. Although laboratories performing DTC tests need to maintain CLIA certification, many DTC tests are not regulated by the US Food and Drug Administration, raising concerns about the accuracy of results. In addition, some testing facilities have claimed exemption from regulatory oversight, asserting that they provide health information and not diagnostic test results. Tandy-Connor and colleagues[21] reported that, of 49 patient samples sent to their clinical diagnostic laboratory (Ambry Genetics) with variants previously identified by DTC laboratories, 40% were false-positive results. Considering the potentially serious implications of genetic testing on patients and their families, false-positive results are a serious concern.

What Do People Do with Results?

Whether accurate or inaccurate, what do consumers do with their results? When faced with an abnormal result, do consumers seek medical care? If the results were false positives, DTC opponents argue that this generates unnecessary physician visits and unnecessary costs to public and private insurers, ultimately leading to increased overall health care costs.[22] Rockwell[22] even argues that, because this risk to patients and the health care system as a whole is so great that state boards should consider sanctions against practitioners who work for DTC testing companies and order testing for consumers without medical history or examination. However, one could just as easily argue that DTC testing helps the health care system. By allowing consumers to screen themselves, they may be able to avoid visits to the doctor's office when their test results are normal.

Kaufman and colleagues[23] conducted an on-line survey of consumers who had used 1 of 3 DTC genetic testing companies. Of the 1048 responders, 43% said they sought additional information about a health condition after testing, 28% discussed their results with a health care professional, 16% changed their medications or supplement regime, and 9% followed up with additional laboratory tests. However, the study could not determine if DTC testing led to improved or worsened outcomes.

Clearly, further studies are needed to quantify the effect of DTC testing on consumers and the health care system as a whole, especially before state boards sanction employees of DTC companies.

Privacy

Privacy is important for all medical testing, but it is of particular importance for genetic testing because of the personal nature of the test results. What assurances can be made by the DTC laboratories regarding confidentiality? Who owns and controls the genetic data? Who should have access to the data? How will patients be protected from improper use? Although the Genetic Information Non-discrimination Act prevents the results of genetic tests from individuals or their family members from impacting access to health insurance and employment, it does not cover life insurance, long-term care, or disability insurance. In addition, there have been high-profile cases of genetic information from DTC companies being used to help law enforcement catch criminals.[24] Are consumers aware of who will have access to their genetic data? Without the requirement for genetic counseling, do consumers understand how the results could impact the privacy of both themselves, and their family members?

JUSTICE

The ethical principle of justice refers to the duty to treat people equally and to fairly allocate benefits, risks, and costs. In recent years there has been an increased focus on health care disparities within the United States. Even for patients with medical coverage, some laboratory testing is not covered fully, or at all, and the cost to the patient may not be apparent until months after testing was performed. One of the attractive features of DTC testing is transparency in cost. Proponents of DTC testing argue that the cost transparency increases accessibility of testing to certain populations. However, some testing, like genetic testing, is expensive, limiting access to those who can afford the cost. Questions arise then about whether DTC genetic testing actually widens the health disparity gap. Few studies have addressed access to DTC testing based on price. In their on-line survey of consumers who had used 1 of 3 DTC genetic testing companies, Kaufman and colleagues[23] noted that the population of responders had high levels of education and income.

The increased use of DTC genetic testing information by law enforcement could affect how consumers perceive the risks and benefits of genetic testing. Perceived risk could increase feelings of distrust or discrimination especially among vulnerable populations such as immigrants, inmates, former convicts, and ethnic minorities.[25,26]

MEDICAL ASSOCIATION STATEMENTS

A number of medical associations have published position statements about DTC testing, however, their viewpoints are far from reaching a consensus. The American Association for Clinical Chemistry suggests that DTC tests should have demonstrated analytical and clinical validity, should be conducted in CLIA-certified laboratories, and should provide sufficient information to assist consumers in ordering and interpreting results.[27] Similarly, the American Society for Clinical Pathology suggests that consumers should select CLIA-certified laboratories and should review results with their physician.[28] The American College of Medical Genetics[29] and American Society For Human Genetics[30] indicate that there should be evidence for the analytical and clinical validity for the genetic testing that is performed, genetic test results should indicate laboratory certification, there should be a health care professional involved in ordering and interpreting genetic, tests and consumers should be informed about what conditions genetic tests can and cannot predict. The American College of Medical Genetics also suggests that privacy should be addressed with consumers regarding who will have access to their genetic test results and leftover DNA.[29] Rafiq and colleagues[31] provide a summary of European guidelines in DTC genetic testing.

In contrast, the College of American Pathologists, an organization of physicians, recommends that laboratory test ordering and interpretation be restricted to physicians.[32] Owing to a lack of consensus, these position statements do little to resolve the ethical questions surrounding DTC laboratory testing.

RECOMMENDATIONS

Clearly, there are a number of ethical concerns surrounding DTC testing. However, surveys indicate that consumers want the ability to order their own laboratory tests (WSJ Survey) and as a result the industry is growing rapidly.[6] What can be done to diminish the ethical concerns surrounding this inevitable change in the health care industry? Improving the quality and oversight of DTC testing could help to balance some of the ethical concerns. Gronowski and colleagues[33] and Lovett and colleagues[20] have proposed actions to improve the reliability and use of DTC medical tests. First, further studies are needed to understand what tests consumers actually order, how test results alter their behavior and the impact of false results (**Box 1**).[20,33] Second, the government should create a DTC formulary. In other words, a list of specific tests that can be ordered by consumers.[20,33] In addition, only tests that have been US Food and Drug Administration approved should be available as DTC testing and the US Food and Drug Administration should be the primary driver for regulation and oversight of DTC testing.[20,33] Third, because the cost of laboratory testing is often what drives people out of mainstream laboratories and into DTC laboratories, more transparency is needed in the cost of laboratory testing.[33] Fourth, as the American Association for Clinical Chemistry and American Society for Clinical Pathology position statements suggest, DTC testing should only be offered by CLIA-certified laboratories.[33] Finally, if more mainstream and reputable laboratories offered DTC testing, some of the concerns about quality

---

Box 1
Recommendations that could help to diminish ethical concerns over DTC testing

Conduct studies to understand what tests consumers order and how the results change their actions

Create a test formulary that outlines which tests can be available DTC

Prohibit non–FDA-approved tests from DTC formularies

The FDA should serve as the primary driver for regulation and oversight

Increase the transparency of laboratory testing costs in all health care settings

DTC testing only from CLIA-certified laboratories

Create DTC testing options from well-respected mainstream laboratories

Increase surveillance of DTC advertising and strict penalties for false advertising

Mandate clear and transparent privacy policies for DTC genetic testing

Mandate pretest and post-test counseling for DTC genetic testing

Medical associations create a consensus position statement

Abbreviation: FDA, US Food and Drug Administration.

of test results could be resolved diminishing the risk of maleficence.[33] We would also suggest several additional actions. First, there should be additional surveillance of DTC advertising and strict penalties for false advertising. Second, we suggest increased oversight of DTC genetic testing, which (1) makes privacy policies clear and transparent and (2) mandates pretest and post-test counseling so that consumers could fully understand the risks, benefits, and limitations of genetic testing. Finally, necessary regulatory changes are more likely to occur if medical associations create a consensus position statement.

SUMMARY

DTC laboratory testing is a rapidly growing sector of health care; however, there are many questions regarding the ethics of allowing consumers to order their own laboratory tests. Although DTC testing would seem to offer autonomy to consumers, autonomy is only maintained if certain criteria are met. In addition, there is little published evidence to support either beneficence or maleficence of DTC testing. Finally, there are conflicting opinions about the justice of DTC testing and whether it increases or decreases health disparities. Clearly, more research is needed to evaluate the effects of DTC testing on the health of consumers and health care as a whole. Here, we provide recommendations for additional actions to improve the reliability and use of DTC medical tests and hence diminish the ethical concerns.

DISCLOSURE

The authors have nothing to disclose.

REFERENCES

1. Kennedy P. Could women be trusted with their own pregnancy tests? New York Times 2016. Available at: https://www.nytimes.com/2016/07/31/opinion/sunday/could-women-be-trusted-with-their-own-pregnancy-tests.html. Accessed July 28, 2019.
2. Romm C. Before there were home pregnancy tests. The Atlantic June 17, 2015. Available at: https://www.theatlantic.com/health/archive/2015/06/history-home-pregnancy-test/396077/. Accessed July 28, 2019.
3. Entwistle PA. Do-it-yourself pregnancy tests: the tip of the iceberg? Am J Public Health 1976;66:1108–9.
4. Arnold C. At-home HIV test poses dilemmas and opportunities. Lancet 2010;380:1045–6.
5. Should consumers be allowed to order their own lab tests? The Wall Street Journal. Available at: https://www.wsj.com/articles/should-consumers-be-allowed-to-order-their-own-lab-tests-1460340176 Accessed July 28, 2019.
6. Kalorama Information Market Intelligence Report. Direct-to-consumer laboratory testing market. 2016. Available at: www.KaloramaInformation.com. Accessed July 28, 2019.
7. Wikipedia. Available at: https://en.wikipedia.org/wiki/Medical_ethics. Accessed July 28, 2019.
8. Gronowski AM, Budelier MM, Campbell SM. Ethics for laboratory medicine. Clin Chem 2019;65:1497–507.
9. Beauchamp TL, Childress JF. Principles of biomedical ethics. 7th edition. New York: Oxford University Press; 2013.

10. American Academy of Pediatrics Policy Statement. Ethical and policy issues in genetic testing and screening of children. Pediatrics 2013;131:620–2.

11. Berg C, Fryer-Edwards K. The ethical challenge of direct-to-consumer genetic testing. J Bus Ethics 2008;77:17–31.

12. Vayena E. Direct-to-consumer genomics on the scales of autonomy. J Med Ethics 2015;41:310–4.

13. Brierley KL, Blouch E, Cogswell W, et al. Adverse events in cancer genetic testing: medical, ethical, legal, and financial implications. Cancer J 2012;18:303–9.

14. Klitzman R, Chung W, Marder K, et al. Attitudes and practices among internists concerning genetic testing. J Genet Couns 2013;22:90–100.

15. U.S. Government Accountability Office. Direct-to-consumer genetic tests: misleading test results are further complicated by deceptive marketing and other questionable practices. Available at: https://www.gao.gov/products/GAO-10-847T. Accessed July 28, 2019.

16. Gollust SE, Hull SC, Wilfond BS. Limitations of direct-to-consumer advertising for clinical genetic testing. JAMA 2002;288:1762–7.

17. Matloff E, Caplan A. Direct to confusion: lessons learned from marketing BRCA testing. Am J Bioeth 2008;8:5–8.

18. Schaper M, Schicktanz S. Medicine, market and communication: ethical considerations in regard to persuasive communication in direct-to-consumer genetic testing services. BMC Med Ethics 2018;19:1–11.

19. Giovanni MA, Fickie MR, Lehmann LS, et al. Health-care referrals from direct-to-consumer genetic testing. Genet Test Mol Biomarkers 2010;14:817–9.

20. Lovett KM, Mackey TK, Liang BA. Evaluating the evidence: direct-to-consumer screening tests. J Med Screen 2012;19:141–53.

21. Tandy-Connor S, Guiltinan J, Krempely K, et al. False-positive results released by direct-to-consumer genetic tests highlight the importance of clinical confirmation testing for appropriate patient care. Genet Med 2018;20:1515–21.

22. Rockwell KL. Direct-to-consumer medical testing in the era of value-based care. JAMA 2017;317:2485–6.

23. Kaufman DJ, Bollinger JM, Dvoskin RL, et al. Risky business: risk perception and use of medical services among customers of DTC personal genetic testing. J Genet Couns 2012;21:413–22.

24. The ethics of catching criminals using their family's DNA. Nature 2018;557:5. Available at: https://www.nature.com/articles/d41586-018-05029-9. Accessed April 1, 2019.

25. Understanding disparities in access to genomic medicine: proceedings of a workshop. The National Academies of Science, Engineering and Medicine. Available at: http://nationalacademies.org/hmd/Activities/Research/GenomicBased Research/2018-JUN-27.aspx. Accessed November 29, 2019.

26. Hendricks-Sturrup RM, Prince AER, Lu CY. Direct-to-consumer genetic testing and potential loopholes in protecting consumer privacy nondiscrimination. JAMA 2019;321:1869–70.

27. American Association for Clinical Chemistry Position Statement. Direct-to-consumer laboratory testing. 2015. Available at: https://www.aacc.org/health-and-science-policy/advocacy/position-statements/2015/direct-to-consumer-laboratory-testing. Accessed July 25, 2019.

28. American Society for Clinical Pathology Policy Statement. Direct access testing. Available at: https://www.ascp.org/content/docs/default-source/policy-statements/ascp-pdft-pp-direct-access-testing.pdf?sfvrsn=2. Accessed July 25, 2019.

29. ACMG Board of Directors. American College of Medical Genetics and Genomics Statement. Direct-to-consumer genetic testing: a revised position statement of the American College of Medical Genetics and Genomics. Genet Med 2016; 18:207–8.
30. ASHG statement on direct-to-consumer genetic testing in the United States A. J Hum Genet 2007;81:635–7.
31. Rafiq M, Ianuale C, Ricciardi W, et al. Direct-to-consumer genetic testing: a systematic review of European guidelines, recommendations and position statements. Genet Test Mol Biomarkers 2015;19:1–13.
32. College of American Pathologists Public Policy. Direct access laboratory testing. Available at: http://webapps.cap.org/apps/docs/statline/pdf/policy_direct_access_laboratory_testing.pdf. Accessed July 25, 2019.
33. Gronowski AM, Haymond S, Master SR. Improving direct-to-consumer medical testing. JAMA 2017;318:1613.

An Overview of Direct-to-Consumer Testing

Nicole V. Tolan, PhD, DABCC

KEYWORDS

- Direct-to-consumer testing • Direct-access testing • Health and wellness monitoring

KEY POINTS

- Insufficient data exist to promote routine wellness monitoring, and there is widespread concern that direct-to-consumer (DTC) testing may provide limited actionable information regarding health and wellness.
- Many DTC testing companies have argued for exemption from clinical diagnostics regulatory oversight, leading to concerns about test quality and the qualifications of testing personnel.
- The same privacy that DTC testing provides, may place patients at greater risk of being lost to follow-up as many have insufficient health literacy to understand their results and seek appropriate follow-up care.
- Most DTC tests have no strong evidence of improved health outcomes and offer no, or negative, value for population-wide screening without sufficient pretest probability of a condition or disease.

INTRODUCTION

Direct-to-consumer (DTC) testing is marketed directly to consumers and consists of laboratory testing performed without a physician's order. DTC testing consists of at-home tests that are available over the counter (OTC) at pharmacy and retail stores, direct-access testing (DAT) that is performed in clinical diagnostic laboratories using in vitro diagnostic (IVD) assays, and recreational genetic and wellness testing available for purchase online and performed by DTC companies.

With changes to the Health Insurance Portability and Accountability Act and the 2014 amendments to the Clinical Laboratory Improvement Act (CLIA) of 1988, patients have the right to access their personal health information.[1] A majority of states also allow for patients to order their own laboratory testing without a physician order, with the exceptions of Connecticut, Georgia, Hawaii, Idaho, Kentucky, New Hampshire, Pennsylvania, Rhode Island, and Tennessee.[2–5] This has led to an increasing number of individuals who are becoming more involved in tracking and managing their own health.

Department of Pathology, Harvard Medical School, Brigham and Women's Hospital, 75 Francis Street, Cotran 2, Boston, MA 02115, USA
E-mail address: ntolan@bwh.harvard.edu

Clin Lab Med 40 (2020) 105–111
https://doi.org/10.1016/j.cll.2019.12.001
0272-2712/20/© 2019 Elsevier Inc. All rights reserved.

labmed.theclinics.com

Laboratory testing results represent a critical element of overall health information and is one of the most frequently accessed areas in the electronic medical record, following widespread adoption of patient portals. Reflecting the public's interest in increased access to this health information, the DTC testing market has seen exponential growth and is projected to surpass $350 million this year.[6] DTC testing also extends to wearable devices, mobile-interfaced devices, and health trackers providing continuous and real-time monitoring, which was valued at more than $13 billion in 2016.[7]

TYPES OF DTC TESTING

Although much of the marketing and many media headlines initially focused on recreational genetics testing, DTC laboratory testing includes any type of test offered directly to consumers that provides an analysis of biological samples, without requiring an order by a health care professional.

Originally, DTC testing comprised US Food and Drug Administration (FDA) or European IVD/CE-marked tests used at home that were available OTC in retail stores or could be purchased on the Internet. OTC tests are defined by the FDA as "tests that can be purchased and used by anyone at home. These do not require a doctor's prescription. If manufacturers intend to sell their test kits OTC, they must demonstrate that untrained lay persons can perform the tests and get good results."[8] A majority of these tests are simple to use and the indications for testing are known to the general public (e.g. human immunodeficiency virus screening, pregnancy testing, and glucose monitoring).[9,10] However, the testing available to consumers has grown significantly more complex with the expansion of DTC testing to include genetic testing and panels of tests advertised for various health assessments and wellness monitoring. The FDA has defined DTC tests as "IVD [assays] that are marketed directly to consumers without the involvement of a health care provider" and state that "these tests generally request the consumer collect a specimen, such as saliva or urine, and send it to the company for testing and analysis."[11] In a several scenarios, samples can be collected and tested by the consumer at home or samples can be collected at regulated phlebotomy collection sites and mailed to a laboratory for testing. With changes in state-level policies that allow DAT,[3] consumers can directly order their own clinical diagnostic testing, composed of screening, monitoring, prognostic, and diagnostic assays typically ordered by physicians for patient care. DAT is performed in the same regulated hospital and commercial clinical diagnostic laboratories as medical testing ordered by a physician and consists of assays reviewed by the FDA or are European CE-marked for IVD testing.

It is becoming increasingly difficult to distinguish the testing performed as DAT, typically performed in CLIA-certified laboratories, from those performed as nondiagnostic DTC testing in unregulated commercial laboratories. Regardless of how samples are collected and testing is performed (**Table 1**), consumers are choosing their own tests and in most cases, receiving their results without the involvement of a physician or other health care professional. Depending on the type of test and its indications for use (recreational in nature or for clinical diagnostic purposes), there are various degrees of oversight by the US FDA, Centers for Medicare and Medicaid Services (CMS), and the Federal Trade Commission (FTC).

CHALLENGES ASSOCIATED WITH DTC TESTING

In today's age of immediate gratification, DTC testing affords consumers accessibility to on-demand and rapid testing without the barriers of the traditional health care

Table 1
Direct-to-consumer testing can be performed for various purposes, with different combinations of sample collection mechanisms and test performance settings, and all with distinctive regulatory oversight requirements
INTENDED USE
Non-Diagnostic in nature: recreational genealogy or inherited traits, wellness monitoring
Clinically informative: genetic risk stratification, chronic disease monitoring, clinical diagnostic direct-access testing
COLLECTION MECHANISM
Sample collection at home:
Fingerstick Capillary Blood
Urine/Fecal
Oral Fluid
Cheek Swab
Sample collection at lab/phlebotomy:
Fingerstick Capillary Blood
Urine/Fecal
Oral Fluid
Cheek Swab
Venipuncture
TESTING MECHANISM
Performed at home:
FDA-cleared OTC testing
Digital health monitoring
Point of collection, non-diagnostic DTC tests
Performed in retail pharmacy or clinic:
CLIA-Waived POC testing (with CLIA certificate of waiver)
Non-diagnostic DTC tests
Mailed to CLIA/non-CLIA laboratory:
CLIA-Waived, moderate and high complexity direct access IVD testing (requires appropriate CLIA certificate)
Diagnostic LDTs (require CLIA certificate and physician order)
Non-Diagnostic DTC LDTs (does not require CLIA certificate, *but should!*)
REGULATORY OVERSIGHT
FDA cleared/approved IVD assays: intended for diagnosis, screening, prognosis, monitoring of disease
Assays not regulated by the FDA: recreational genetics, wellness testing, and digital health monitoring
CMS oversight of CLIA-certified laboratories: maintain quality system practices to ensure accuracy through inspections and participation in PT surveys
All DTC testing marketing is subject to FTC requirements: ensuring against false claims and deceptive marketing practices

system, namely a health care provider. Proponents of DTC testing often tout the increase in wellness monitoring fundamentally allows for detection of changes in health and the ability to detect and monitor disease sooner and more robustly than what typically is done through a physician's office visit.[11] In this era of quantified self-monitoring and wellness monitoring, wearables offer the benefits of real-time alerts. Critics warn consumers, however, of excessive tendencies that lead to the worried well.[12]

Questionable Health Care Value and Quality

There is similar, widespread concern that DTC testing may provide limited actionable information regarding individual health and wellness. Insufficient data exist to demonstrate that frequent monitoring against one's own baseline provides improved health outcomes. In addition, the frequency of testing and reasonable intervals for monitoring have not yet been demonstrated.

Health systems and federal agencies, namely CMS, have implemented various checks and balances to improve adherence to evidence-based testing guidelines (eg, pay-for-performance reimbursement models) and prevent unnecessary testing (prohibited bundled testing) in the fee-for-service environment of clinical diagnostic testing. These same regulations, however, have not been put in place to protect those consumers performing DTC testing. In fact, panels of tests for various health monitoring purposes are the primary focus of DTC testing companies. DTC testing companies are not subject to these same efforts to reduce high-volume, low-value clinical testing, which are further complicated by deceptive marketing practices.[13,14]

Regulatory Considerations

Regulated clinical diagnostic laboratories are required to maintain compliance with certain quality assurance measures, such as thorough education and competency documentation, biannual inspection, and participation in external quality assurance and proficiency testing (PT) surveys. These CLIA regulatory requirements are enforced by CMS and agencies with deemed status to ensure high-quality testing and, ultimately, test accuracy. Several DTC testing companies have claimed exemption, however, from these same regulations, arguing that they are not providing diagnostic test results. The majority of DTC testing has not been considered clinical diagnostic testing by regulatory bodies, such as the FDA, and has not been regulated as such, as long as these companies do not provide results analysis or medical advice pertaining to the diagnosis, treatment, or management of disease.[15] This lack of regulatory oversight has led, however, to concerns regarding test quality and the training/credentials of testing personnel.[16] With reduced quality assurance comes an increased inherent risk of unnecessary stress and consumers acting on inaccurate results.[17] This is particularly true for consumers performing DTC testing and making health management decisions, including modifying their medications, without a health care provider involved.[2]

Breakdown in Communication

All medical testing performed in clinical diagnostic laboratories requires several result recording and notification mechanisms, including critical call-backs to patients' health care providers and reporting of certain conditions to local, state, and federal agencies. DTC testing affords patients added privacy and control over who their testing results are shared with; however, this model directly opposes the efforts of integrated health care delivery and data integration through a universal health record. Furthermore, these consumers are at greater risk of being lost to follow-up due to the breakdown of communication with a health care provider, especially in the absence of sufficient health literacy to understand and follow-up with their test results, as detailed (see Daniel T. Holmes's article, "Self-Ordering Laboratory Testing: Limitations When a Physician Isn't Part of the Model," and Nicole V. Tolan's article, "Health Literacy and the Desire to Manage One's Own Health," in this issue).

The Costs of Privacy

Although it is understandable that consumers desire privacy pertaining to sexually transmitted infectious disease testing, health care providers do not have the opportunity to consult patients on additional testing that may be required or warn consumers of their risks of spreading infection and ways to mitigate that risk. Although the Genetic Information Nondiscrimination Act (2008) protects some individuals from health insurance and employment discrimination based on genetic testing results, consumers may voluntarily make their health information public, even sharing on social media platforms, which may have unforeseen consequences for consumers as well as their biological relatives.

Downstream Effects

Increased access to testing, when appropriate testing is performed, can be particularly beneficial for patients who have high deductible/catastrophic insurance or are uninsured. However, many of the tests offered by DTC testing companies are advertised as lifestyle testing and offer no, or negative, value for population-wide screening without strong evidence of improved health outcomes.[4,18] Low-risk individuals without sufficient pre-test probability, who would otherwise be identified through physician examination and review of clinical history and symptoms, are at greater risk of receiving inaccurate results (false positive or false negative), which are likely to initiate a cascade of additional, unnecessary follow-up testing from their health care provider.[19]

Although DTC testing itself is relatively inexpensive and paid out-of-pocket by the consumer, all downstream health care costs are billed to insurers, who may or may not pay for follow-up services, considering a physician did not initiate the DTC testing. In this way, the DTC testing companies are not subject to the same clinical diagnostic testing regulations as are health care systems and providers.

FINAL THOUGHTS

There are inherent risks associated with purchasing unregulated medical devices online.

For example, in April 2019, the FDA put out a safety communication warning the public from purchasing test strips (used for glucose testing or coagulation monitoring) online that were not authorized for sale in the United States. These included not only strips without clearance/approval from the FDA but also strips that were previously purchased, and potentially *used*, by another consumer. These strips carry the potential risk of infection through blood and biological fluid contamination, inaccurate test results from incorrect handling/storage, modified or concealed expiration dates, or unknown tampering with strips—potentially leading to serious injury or death.[20]

It is becoming more and more difficult to trace where products are coming from and if DTC testing is provided from a reputable source. Without strict regulatory oversight, these same risks also could apply to the providers of DTC testing.

Federal and state agencies need to provide sufficient oversight of the DTC testing market, including the requirement for testing to be performed in CLIA-certified laboratories. Inspection of commercial laboratories is required to ensure test quality and validity of test results (eg, quality-control measures to maintain accuracy throughout the testing cycle). Increased surveillance by the FTC is required to protect consumers from deceptive marketing practices with particular focus on how the results are impacting consumers and the traditional health care system tasked with follow-up testing.

DISCLOSURE

The author has nothing to disclose.

REFERENCES

1. Centers for Medicare and Medicaid Services. CLIA program and HIPAA privacy rule; patients' access to test reports. Federal Register. 2014. Available at: https://

www.federalregister.gov/documents/2014/02/06/2014-02280/clia-program-and-hipaa-privacy-rule-patients-access-to-test-reports. Accessed August 1, 2019.

2. American Association for Clinical Chemistry. Position statement: direct-to-consumer laboratory testing. 2015. Available at: https://www.aacc.org/-/media/Files/Health-and-Science-Policy/Position-Statements/DirecttoConsumerLaboratoryTesting.pdf?la=en&hash=18864E273BDECF27DFE2F3305E21422AD1BB8A22. Accessed August 1, 2019.

3. Alltucker Ken. Tech company Theranos pushes consumer lab-testing bill. The Republic. 2013. Available at: http://www.azcentral.com/story/news/arizona/politics/2015/02/27/%20high-tech-pushes-consumer-friendly-lab-%20testing/24150229/. Accessed August 1, 2019.

4. Rockwell KL. Direct-to-consumer medical testing in the era of value-based care. JAMA 2017;317:2485–6.

5. American Society for Clinical Laboratory Science. Direct Access Testing. Position paper: consumer access to laboratory testing and information. 2012. Available at: https://www.ascls.org/position-papers/179-direct-access-testing/155-direct-access-testing. Accessed August 1, 2019.

6. The market for direct-to-consumer genetic testing and routine laboratory testing. Kalorama Information. Available at: http://www.kaloramainformation.com/Direct-Consumer-DTC-9588755/. Accessed August 1, 2019.

7. The market for wearable devices, Kalorama Information. Available at: http://www.kaloramainformation.com/Wearable-Devices-10376869/. Accessed August 1, 2019.

8. US Food and Drug Administration. Home use tests: glossary. 2017. Available at: https://www.fda.gov/medical-devices/home-use-tests/home-use-tests-glossary#:~:targetText=Over%2DThe%2DCounter(OTC,used%20by%20anyone%20at%20home.&targetText=Qualitative%20Test%3A%20A%20test%20that,the%20person%20has%20the%20condition. Accessed August 1, 2019.

9. Gronowski AM, Haymond S, Master SR. Improving direct-to-consumer medical testing. JAMA 2017;318:1613.

10. US Food and Drug Administration. Direct-to-Consumer Tests. 2018. Available at: https://www.fda.gov/medical-devices/vitro-diagnostics/direct-consumer-tests. Accessed August 1, 2019.

11. Ajana B. Digital health and the biopolitics of the quantified self. Digit Health 2017; 3:1–18.

12. Welch HG, Schwartz L, Woloshin S. Overdiagnosed: making people sick in the pursuit of health. Beacon Press; 2011.

13. Neighmond. U.S. Justice Department charges 35 people in Fraudulent genetic testing scheme. Shots Health News from NPR. 2019. Available at: https://www.npr.org/sections/health-shots/2019/09/27/765230011/u-s-justice-department-charges-35-people-in-fraudulent-genetic-testing-scheme. Accessed October 17, 2019.

14. General Accountability Office. Direct-to-consumer genetic tests: misleading test results are further complicated by deceptive marketing and other questionable practices. GAO-10-847T. 2010. Available at: https://www.gao.gov/products/%20GAO-10-847T. Accessed August 1, 2019.

15. McGuire AL, Burke W. Healthsystem implications of direct-to-consumer personal genome testing. Public Health Genomics 2011;14(1):53–8.

16. General Accountability Office. Nutrigenetic testing: tests purchased from four web sites mislead consumers. GAO-06-977T. 2006. Available at: http://www.gao.gov/products/GAO-06-977T. Accessed August 1, 2019.

17. Lippi G, Favaloro EJ, Plebani M. Direct-to-consumer testing: more risks than opportunities. Int J Clin Pract 2011;65:1221–9.
18. Lovett KM, Mackey TK, Liang BA. Evaluating the evidence: direct-to-consumer screening tests advertised online. J Med Screen 2012;19(3):141–53.
19. Kaufman DJ, Bollinger JM, Dvoskin RL, et al. Risky business: risk perception and the use of medical services among customers of DTC personal genetic testing. J Genet Couns 2012;21(3):413–22.
20. US Food and Drug Administration. The FDA Warns Against Use of Previously Owned Test Strips or Test Strips Not Authorized for Sale in the United States: FDA Safety Communication. 2019. Available at: https://www.fda.gov/medical-devices/safety-communications/fda-warns-against-use-previously-owned-test-strips-or-test-strips-not-authorized-sale-united-states. Accessed August 1, 2019.

Moving?

Make sure your subscription moves with you!

To notify us of your new address, find your **Clinics Account Number** (located on your mailing label above your name), and contact customer service at:

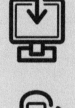

Email: **journalscustomerservice-usa@elsevier.com**

800-654-2452 (subscribers in the U.S. & Canada)
314-447-8871 (subscribers outside of the U.S. & Canada)

Fax number: **314-447-8029**

Elsevier Health Sciences Division
Subscription Customer Service
3251 Riverport Lane
Maryland Heights, MO 63043

*To ensure uninterrupted delivery of your subscription, please notify us at least 4 weeks in advance of move.